"In *Personal Grief Rituals*, Paul Martin has produced that rarest of things in the literature on grief therapy: a compendium that is at once deeply scholarly while being immensely practical. Chapter after chapter, I found myself intrigued, instructed and inspired by his astonishing and appreciative grasp of the endless cultural variations on rituals of mourning, while counterbalancing this with a theoretically sophisticated and empirically informed psychodynamic understanding of the nuances of grieving that collective practices often only awkwardly accommodate. Drawing with equal alacrity on classical attachment theory and contemporary models of coping with loss, Martin then proceeds to offer clear and helpful principles for co-constructing with clients healing rituals of both remembrance and release, conveyed by concrete and relatable case studies. For its recognition of the dialectics of honoring continuing bonds while also embracing life, and its balanced critique of the siren song of endless mourning and a defensive deafness to the natural call of grief, I recommend this infectiously readable volume to every grief therapist who seeks to transcend words alone to help clients reach beyond loss to life, and to embrace the meaning that can be found in mourning."

Robert A. Neimeyer, *editor of* New Techniques of Grief Therapy *and director of Portland Institute for Loss and Transition*

"This is a highly valuable and thought-provoking book, a leading-edge contribution to understanding a critically important topic in bereavement research and practice, namely, the role of rituals in adapting to the death of someone close. It offers a fresh approach, drawing on the author's remarkably broad knowledge in the fields of sociology, cultural anthropology and psychology, to argue the case for creating personal grief rituals when established ones fail to facilitate healthy grieving. This he does by inter-weaving descriptions of rituals throughout history and around the world with his understanding of the relevant psychological literature, as well as by drawing on his own clinical skill and experience. In doing so, he links theory with application, demonstrating how therapists may help bereaved clients with grieving difficulties, through designing individually tailored rituals in accordance with the person's specific experience and needs. In my view, the book's appeal will be far-reaching both within and beyond the field of thanatology."

Margaret Stroebe, *professor emerita at the Department of Clinical and Health Psychology, Utrecht University, and the Department of Clinical Psychology and Experimental Psychopathology, Groningen University*

"Paul Martin's *Personal Grief Rituals* is a fascinating exploration of the role of rituals in grief and mourning. Artfully blending insights from anthropology, psychology, history, and sociology, *Personal Grief Rituals* is an amazing asset to death educators, counselors, and the general public. It is bound to become a classic work!"

Kenneth J. Doka, *senior vice-president for Grief Programs, the Hospice Foundation of America; professor emeritus, the College of New Rochelle*

Personal Grief Rituals

Personal Grief Rituals presents a new model for how bereaved individuals can create unique expressions of mourning that are tailored to their psychological needs and grounded in memories and emotions specific to the relationship they lost.

This book examines cultures across the world and throughout history to shed light on how humanity has always turned to grief rituals and how custom can stifle one's pursuit of healthy and meaningful mourning. Contemporary psychological research, most notably attachment theory, provides an in-depth understanding of how each individual's subjective experience of loss varies and why complicated bereavement may emerge. Richly detailed psychotherapy case studies exemplify innovative strategies for designing personal grief rituals. Where one person may visit an old haunt to express sorrow, another might use symbols to strengthen their connection to the deceased, and still another could cast aside vestiges of the past.

Personal Grief Rituals is an excellent resource for professionals, students studying the psychology of loss, or anyone hoping to carve a new path through their own grief and mourning.

Paul M. Martin is a licensed clinical psychologist, the assistant director of the Center for Grief Recovery, and an adjunct professor at Northwestern University. He specializes in psychotherapy for those struggling with complicated bereavement and regularly provides continuing education workshops and individual consultation for professionals.

Personal Grief Rituals

Creating Unique Expressions of Loss and Meaningful Acts of Mourning in Clinical or Private Settings

Paul M. Martin

Routledge
Taylor & Francis Group
LONDON AND NEW YORK

Cover image: Artwork by Kurt Fondriest, Expressive art therapist

First published 2023
by Routledge
4 Park Square, Milton Park, Abingdon, Oxon OX14 4RN

and by Routledge
605 Third Avenue, New York, NY 10158

Routledge is an imprint of the Taylor & Francis Group, an informa business

British Library Cataloguing-in-Publication Data
A catalogue record for this book is available from the British Library

Library of Congress Cataloging-in-Publication Data
A catalog record for this book has been requested

ISBN: 978-0-815-38411-3 (hbk)
ISBN: 978-0-815-38412-0 (pbk)
ISBN: 978-1-351-20487-3 (ebk)

DOI: 10.4324/9781351204873

Typeset in Garamond
by Apex CoVantage, LLC

This book is dedicated to anyone who lost a loved one in the early throes of the COVID-19 pandemic, was left to mourn in isolation, and did not know what to do with their grief while alone and separated from their usual supports and cultural customs.

Contents

Acknowledgments

First of all, I wish to express the immense love and appreciation I have for my wife, Ashlie, whose undying love and encouragement buoyed me over the past six years as I wrote this book. I look forward to penning the next one with her by my side to share in its joys and frustrations. We are lucky to have two wonderful children, each of whom have taught me more about psychology than any book or journal article ever could. My relationships with them have taken shape during the duration of this project and have shown me both the awe-inspiring power of forging close bonds as well as the importance of giving our most cherished attachments ample space to grow.

I owe a special debt of gratitude to David Fireman, director of the Center for Grief Recovery. This book owes its existence to him taking me under his wing when I was fresh out of graduate school and giving me the opportunity to do meaningful and varied work with bereaved clientele across Chicago while fulfilling the center's mission: *to empower individuals to heal and enrich their own lives*. I am indebted to the patients I have worked with for entrusting me with their stories and their well-being as they faced tremendous hardships; the lessons I have learned from witnessing such resiliency and creativity have colored the pages of this project. And to the many students and fellow professionals I have had the pleasure to teach, I am grateful for their curiosity and thought-provoking questions, all of which invited me to articulate my amorphous musings about loss, grief, and mourning into a book that now has a definitive form.

I want to give thanks to Kate Hawes, who first agreed to take on this project many years ago and waited patiently across the pond as I learned, in piecemeal, how to prepare a professional manuscript for publication. This book would have never come to pass without her generosity and guidance along the way.

Also, I have been blessed again and again to find myself in the company of colleagues, dear friends, and loving family members who were there to lend a boost to my morale when I needed it the most. To those who kept me positive and inquired into my progress with a calm smile, you know who you are. A celebratory toast is in order!

And finally, I would like to pay tribute to all three of my parents, who somehow managed to instill within me the absurd notion that I can accomplish whatever I set out to do with my life. Thank you.

Chapter 1

Cultural grief rituals and the mourning process

An anthropological perspective

Somewhere in India, a young man listens to the crackling of his father's funeral pyre and waits for confirmation that the skull, having been subjected to immense heat, has finally split open. In Mexico, generations of the living, both young and old, share a meal with the dead at a gravesite. A village of people in Ghana readies themselves to bury a member of their community in a coffin fashioned to look like a bowling pin, or a remodeled car, or whatever hobby the deceased once enjoyed. In Japan, a woman shares family news with her great-grandmother who passed away decades prior. And on the islands of Hawaii, immediately after the bereaved have finished washing and dressing the deceased's body, a chorus of screams and wailing reverberates out from the home to signal to all within earshot that death has arrived.

Each of these grief rituals, however different from one another, is surely felt to be the appropriate course of mourning for most members of the culture that subscribes to them. But just as any group of people in any corner of the world may find their neighbor's customs odd and unfamiliar, so too does the errant individual within a community find themselves participating in death rites that, although occurring in their native land, feel alien to them, as if spoken in a foreign tongue. The individual utters insincere words. They partake in dances whose movements fail to resonate. They emote inauthentic feelings of anger or sorrow purely for show. They bid farewell when they have not yet truly let go, and they hold on to the deceased's presence when they would rather cut ties.

It gives me great joy to envisage those individuals stealing away in quiet solitude, free from the scrutinizing gaze of others, to shake off the dust of stale ceremonies and enact more meaningful and personal expressions of their grief. Perhaps they will burn an effigy or cast a symbol of the deceased into a body of water. They may visit an old haunt to converse with the dead once more . . . or to say goodbye. The bereaved might even let loose a furtive smile of relief or cry tears that custom had forbidden. Whatever symbolic and expressive actions the individual creates for themselves away from the constraints of tradition, my hope is that their experience of loss and

DOI: 10.4324/9781351204873-1

mourning comes to feel truer as a result of its performance, and that greater voice is given to the unique thoughts and feelings about the relationship they lost, thoughts and feelings which the collective zeitgeist of culture could never understand.

Grief rituals across time and space: A brief history of how humans have mourned

Death renders the human animal restless. Compelled to act, we seem to be incapable of standing by idly amid the chaos of grief and the blinding glare of mortality. This impulse to actively take part in the process of gracefully relinquishing our bonds precedes recorded history. It has always resided within us.

Since time immemorial, humankind has banded together and developed elaborate rituals to mourn the dead. Our ancestors left behind clues that evidence ongoing efforts to contemplate an afterlife and grapple with how to aid the soul in its transition from one plane of existence to the next and, in turn, how to help ourselves transition through the process of letting go. As far back as 60,000 BC, Neanderthal burial grounds have been decorated with animal antlers and flower fragments placed near the body. Ancient Egyptians, circa 2600 BC, developed embalming techniques and practiced mummification to preserve bodies of their deceased and facilitate transmigration of the soul into the afterlife. The ancient Greeks' rituals took an interesting turn around 800 BC. As both preservation of the corpse and burial in the ground fell out of favor, the Greeks opted for cremation on funeral pyres; smoke and ash lifted the soul in its ascent towards the heavens. Evidence has been found dating back to AD 7 that Native Americans started burying their dead with gifts and goods such as tools and jewelry, akin to the Egyptians' similar efforts to prepare their deceased for the next world.

Just as grief rituals have centered on processes for letting go and embracing absence, humans have also used ritual for the sake of holding on to the dead and facilitating symbolic access to their loved ones' continued presence. *Sosen-suhai*, or ancestor worship, became commonplace in China during the Shang Dynasty sometime between 1523 and 1028 BC. Still in practice throughout China and Japan to this day, a system of rituals allows surviving family members ongoing connection and communication with departed family members. Circa AD 1500, the Aztecs began celebrating *Dia de los Muertos*, or Day of the Dead, as a means by which they, too, could keep the spirits of their ancestors alive and present. And in recent years, people have begun launching cremated remains of their loved ones into space to be dispersed among the stars. Not unlike a bereaved individual who gravitates towards visiting a grave site in hopes of reviving a sense of their loved one's presence, some now do the same by looking up at the stars.

Grief rituals redefined: What they are and what they are not

Empathic communication may uplift the bereaved for a moment, and platitudes may soothe the pain of loss for a short time, but reliance upon mere word-bound interventions ultimately fails to plumb the depths of grief. Embodied responses to loss are needed in order to facilitate the complex and multifaceted processes of mourning. Humankind has long turned to the organized patterns of behavior within rituals to give palpable expression to the deep wells of grief, to release earthly ties with the deceased in acts of catharsis, to re-establish order after the deceased's absence tears a hole in the fabric of community, and to concretize the ongoing symbolic presence of loved ones after they are gone.

And yet many people have deep misgivings about the potential benefits of such. Merely uttering *ritual* is sure to raise a few eyebrows, as the word itself carries a host of misunderstandings and negative connotations. For some, ritual evokes images of strange ceremonies carried out in the dark by religious zealots, of peculiar efforts to wield fire and sorcery to exert control over fate, or of barbaric and superstitious animal sacrifices to the gods. The fields of psychology and psychiatry have seemed to reduce ritual to the pathological and maladaptive behaviors associated with obsessive-compulsive disorder: mundane and repetitive compulsions – excessive handwashing, for example – that serve the defensive function of keeping cognition, memory, and emotion at bay. Even the colloquial use of *ritual* in everyday vernacular denotes a rigid and mechanized routine to be carried out with minimal thought or reflection for the sole purpose of ensuring efficient time management. But it is precisely these psychological elements of emotion, introspection, meaning, and memory that are to be awakened within grief rituals. Traditionally, grief rituals have consisted of carefully planned social gatherings designed to encourage the bereaved to be present with the intensity of their feelings, to express their yearning for reunion, to move forward with intention and meaning, and to contemplate where the deceased's spirit will reside. Grief rituals are anything but perfunctory routines.

Ritual can be plainly defined as "a solemn ceremony consisting of a series of actions performed according to a prescribed order" (Lexico, n.d.). While this definition highlights the importance of predetermined and organized behaviors, its affective range is too narrow, suggesting that the emotional experience of ritual consists only of that which is grave and somber. Therese Rando (1985), a clinical psychologist specializing in issues related to loss and grief, has offered a more open and profound definition of ritual: "a specific behavior or activity which gives symbolic expression to certain feelings and thoughts of the actor" (p. 236). With Rando's definition, we begin to appreciate that grief rituals use organized action to evoke *a multitude of potential emotions and cognitions* pertaining to the individual's subjective experience of loss and mourning. Anger, relief, sadness, anxiety, or joy all have the potential to color a ritual's performance. Furthermore, Rando recognized the importance of symbolism in acts of grief and mourning; audible words and observable gestures external to the bereaved represent that which is internal and give shape to what is otherwise inchoate and nebulous. Laird (1984) spoke of how symbolic representation in rituals provides a means by which the nonverbal aspects of the self and one's most important relationships can be expressed, organized, and integrated along with those aspects that are more overtly verbal.

But there is one more important piece to consider: *meaning-making*. Grief rituals involve more than the use of behaviors and symbols to manifest latent thoughts and feelings about a loss. Schnell (2009) has conceptualized rituals as formalized patterns of behavior that help construct meaning around a personally relevant event. They may very well be designed to fit within preexisting structures of meaning about death, subsequent grief, and the process of mourning, but according to Robert Neimeyer's (2002) constructivist perspective, loss often challenges the bereaved to reconstruct core beliefs and assumptions one uses to make sense of the world after a loss, to make meaning anew and rebuild that which death has torn down.

This constellation of ideas from Rando, Laird, Schnell, and Neimeyer coalesces to form a more robust portrait of all that a grief ritual entails: *a specific series of actions, grounded in meaning about death and mourning, that gives symbolic expression to thoughts and feelings about a particular loss.* This revised definition affords the freedom to see *personal grief rituals* as something that can be created to cater to the individual's needs and subjective experience of loss. The unique thoughts, meaning-making, and feelings of the ritual's actor can then be represented in action. Personal grief rituals may be most important in instances when culture has not provided sufficient opportunity for such. But before we consider how the individual can break away from what culture prescribes, we turn to the study of cultural anthropology and endeavor to understand what cultures around the world aim to facilitate with their particular brand of grief rituals.

The many functions of cultural grief rituals

A survey of cultures throughout the world reveals a wide array of forms that grief rituals can take. The great variety of actions performed, as well as the broad range of emotional timbre that comes forth as a result, makes evident that ritual serves myriad functions for different peoples. First of all, the bereaved are afforded *an opportunity to express emotions*. Affects as disparate as sadness, joy, and anger find an outlet in a social context and within a circumscribed duration of time. The American funeral is marked by a solemn display of sorrow (Metcalf & Huntington, 1991). Australian Aborigines embody the raw anger of grief through acts of self-injury (Farrelly & Francis, 2009). And the Zulu people of South Africa, particularly younger generations, encourage expressions of joy and zeal for life after the initial funeral as they gather to listen to music and dance through the night during an *after-tears party* (Abruzzini, 2017).

On a most practical level, Birx (2006) observed that grief rituals help *determine how the body is to be handled.* Interment of the deceased beneath the ground in a burial ceremony remains a common practice around the globe, and a great many cultures find immense value in washing the body soon after death. Whereas the ancient Egyptians relied upon mummification to dispose of the corpse, the Vikings and the ancient Greeks came to prefer cremation, still widely used by modern-day Hindus and peoples of Bali.

Many cultures' rituals center on some form of secondary burial, a prolonged process during which the body is buried only to be exhumed after many years have lapsed, at which point the remains are managed as seen fit and laid to rest in their final interment. Secondary burials hinge upon differing beliefs about when the moment of death truly arrives. These grief rituals and others that involve handling corporeal remains highlight the additional importance of *actualizing the reality of a loss.*

The sight of a body lying still in a coffin. The sounds of family members weeping. The looks of sympathy in the eyes of friends and family. The familiarity of funeral rites and symbols of mourning specific to one's culture. Such visual and audible cues drive home the stark reality that someone has died. So crucial in facilitating a healthy mourning process, grief rituals of all kinds provide this straightforward confrontation with the blunt truth of death and stillness. Even the tradition of holding a wake with an open casket has its roots in Ireland's efforts to ensure that the dead are resolutely gone and not mistakenly buried alive (Grainger, 1998).

Some communities use grief rituals not only to confirm the passing of one of its members but also to provide *an opportunity to say goodbye to the deceased,* what Van der Hart and Ebbers (1981) referred to as a "rite of separation" (p. 190). In the Sanyuan Village of China, those who are moments away from their last breath are held upright near an open window; any kin of a dying parent is compelled to use this precise moment to say goodbye and part ways. By bidding farewell to the dead, the bereaved decidedly distance themselves from the past (Chen, 2000). Thus, grief rituals also serve to *mark a transition in time* that demarcates what had come before and what lies ahead. Romanoff and Terenzio (1998) stated that one of the most important functions of funerals is their ability to provide a clear sense of transition that propels the living towards the future. Those in the Philippines regularly practice a death anniversary ritual, during which the bereaved burn nonvaluable belongings of the dead to symbolize that formal mourning has been drawn to a close and that it is time to embrace new life once again (Santiago, 1993).

Kenneth Doka (2012) stated that rituals simultaneously mark a transition in the bereaved individual's journey through grief and mourning while also *facilitating the spirit's journey to the afterlife*. The Egyptians, like so many civilizations throughout history, centered their death rites and rituals around a belief in transmigration of the soul, and the Tibetan ritual of a sky burial, in which the corpse is picked clean by carrion-eaters that proceed skyward towards the heavens, underscores the importance for many of ensuring the deceased's ascension to a new plane of existence.

Just as rituals promote a transition away from earthly ties, they can also help to *establish and maintain an ongoing symbolic connection to the deceased*. Romanoff and Terenzio (1998) highlight *continuation* as an essential function of ritual. And proponents of *continuing bonds* theory certainly echo this notion (Goss & Klass, 2005; Klass et al., 1996; Worden, 2008). Lewis-Williams and Pearce (2005) have argued that prehistoric tombs served as places to revisit the dead and maintain an ongoing relationship. Ancestor worship in China perpetuates meaningful ties to the dead over many years and across generations. The Mexican holiday of Dia de los Muertos puts aside time each year to coax out spirits of the dead and for families to celebrate life alongside the felt presence of their departed loved ones.

In a slight variation on this theme that entails acknowledging reality and establishing an ongoing connection, Doka (2012) gives special consideration to "rituals of affirmation" (p. 342) that maintain continuity beyond the moment of death and *validate a relationship or the legacy of the deceased*. Muslims strive to perform good deeds in memory of their dead (Yasien-Esmael & Rubin, 2005). The Ojibwe, a Native American tribe of indigenous people living in Canada and the northern regions of the United States, hold an annual feast to nourish the mourners and honor the dead by regaling one another with fond memories of those they have lost (Walker-Gillet, 2011). Indeed, funeral rituals and mourning customs around the world are often used to stimulate memories of loved ones and ensure that the deceased's legacy lives on.

The task model of mourning

The various functions of grief rituals described above converge around four central themes that align with William Worden's (2008) *task model of mourning*, which posits that the journey of mourning is successfully traversed only insofar as the bereaved manage four separate but interdependent goals, or tasks. And he is certainly not the only psychologist to insist upon the importance of what the bereaved must do in order to mourn. Therese Rando's own model, the *six-R processes of mourning* (Rando, 1993), complements Worden's and further emphasizes a distinction between the passive experience of what is felt amid grief and the need to respond to loss with an active stance. Grief rituals from every corner of the world provide its participants with the means to approach one or more of these essential tasks.

Task I: To accept the reality of the loss

The bereaved are quite aware of the stark truth that someone important to them has died. Emptiness echoes in every room they enter. Final moments with the deceased linger in the survivor's mind as the pallor of death haunts their memories. And yet disbelief persists and proves to be fiercely tenacious throughout mourning. Denial of the finality of loss is an albatross that hangs over every feeling of grief and every memory about the deceased. Task I in Worden's model emphasizes how imperative it is that the bereaved endeavor to unburden themselves of denial and accept reality in all its harshness. Similarly, Rando's model highlights the crucial processes of overcoming avoidance of reality in order to *recognize the loss* and the importance of confronting it by means of *relinquishing old attachments*. Those rituals that dictate "how the body is handled," that "actualize the loss," and those that "provide an opportunity to say goodbye to the deceased" while also "facilitating the soul's journey" all underscore the crucial importance of acknowledging death and the subsequent absence of a once-present relationship.

Task II: To process the pain of grief

Worden and Rando both acknowledge that the emotional component of grief arises spontaneously within the bereaved. Survivors of loss have little say over the intensity of feelings that besiege them. Still, they are encouraged to assume a degree of control and actively express their pain in whatever form and intensity it assumes, be it sadness, anger, fear, or happiness. Rando speaks of *reacting to the separation* as one way to directly confront the emotional reaction to loss. Rituals that "facilitate the expression of emotions" allow the bereaved to embrace complex feelings and acknowledge discomfort stemming from all that has been lost after death has torn away an important relationship.

Task III: To adjust to a world without the deceased

Sigmund Freud (1917) once quipped that the state of mourning is characterized by a feeling that the world has been rendered empty. Indeed, in the aftermath of a death, roles once filled by the deceased are left vacant, highlighting their absence in the home and the community. Familiar meals do not get cooked. Positions of leadership go unmanned and leave many without proper guidance as the ships of community service and business careen off course. Sources of emotional support and comfort are suddenly unavailable. Within the six-R process model, *readjusting to the world without forgetting* addresses the need for families and entire communities to reassign responsibilities and for individuals to become comfortable within their new roles.

There are also, according to Worden, internal and spiritual adjustments to be made as the bereaved orient themselves to alterations in identity and belief systems. Survivors of loss benefit from allowing themselves to care about new relationships and activities, thus accommodating changes to life in the deceased's absence, what Rando referred to as *reinvesting new energy*. This task emphasizes all that is new and uncharted after a loss, and so those rituals that "mark a transition" and demarcate a moment in time are essential in that they signal the need for change to follow. Further, those rituals that "facilitate the soul's journey," referenced above in connection to Task I, also encourage the bereaved to move forward as well and leave the past where it belongs.

Task IV: To find an enduring connection with the deceased in the midst of embarking on a new life

To mourn is to embrace paradox. The bereaved fix their eyes on a future ahead but pause to gaze back into the past. They sit around the dinner table and forge new memories with family and friends while rekindling reminiscences of those whom they dined with before. Mourning, it seems, is most robust when simultaneously letting go and holding on. Worden's model not only permits ongoing ties to the memory of those who have been lost, but its fourth task also accentuates just how imperative it is to remain tethered to our history even as we walk away from it. It is paramount to both recalibrate to the reality of a new world without the deceased and feel genuinely connected to what came before. This abstract and subjective sense of felt presence provides many with a semblance of comfort that continues to satiate relational and emotional needs. Rando's theory compels the bereaved to *recollect and re-experience*, as remembrance offers an important avenue towards maintaining a meaningful bond with our departed loved ones, if only on a representational level, for the remainder of our days. Grief rituals that "establish ongoing connections" to the dead and "validate their legacy" help strengthen crucial ties to one's most cherished relationships even in their absence.

The problem of interpretation: Assumed uniformity and the cultural other

From the celebrations of Dia de los Muertos in Mexico, to the precise timing with which Hindus cremate their dead, to the delayed secondary burials still in practice among the Malagasy of Madagascar, the Choctaw Native Americans of Oklahoma, and the Ifugao people of the Philippines, the sprawling assortment of cultural grief rituals is awe-inspiring. It can be dizzying to consider how one culture's actions and their underlying systems of meaning are in stark contrast with another's. Traditional death rites are tailored to fit within the dominant belief systems of a culture and to meet the unique psychological needs of its people. As follows, questions about how to mourn will be answered in markedly different ways: Is the emotional component of grief to be expressed openly or contained? And which specific feeling states are appropriate? Which are to be discouraged? Are the body and soul to be relinquished through burial, natural decay in the open air, or fire? Should the bereaved disposed of the body sooner or later? Is there any room in mourning for an ongoing, symbolic connection to the dead . . . or should ties to the deceased be cleaved off? What signifies an adaptive transition away from the past and into a future without the deceased?

Such variance between different groups of people tempts us to conclude that certain cultures have grasped how to traverse the mourning process, whereas others' customs and beliefs must surely be leading the bereaved astray. But lo and behold, no singular correct path emerges. And therein lies the value and utility in Worden's task model. His quadrant of tasks provides a system through which we can begin to interpret the meaning behind a grief ritual in terms of its specific focal point and the psychological needs it deems most important. Where one cultures' customs may emphasize the need to maintain an ongoing connection to the deceased (Task IV), another will use rituals to tend more to the importance of recognizing the reality of a loss (Task I) and adapting to life without the deceased (Task III). And still another will have developed sequences of behavior that give expression to specific pangs of grief (Task II). Each culture's efforts to cope with and make meaning out of loss facilitate some strand of the multifaceted web that is the mourning process.

A far-reaching survey of death rites and rituals around the world illuminates the nuances of mourning we may share with even our most remote neighbors. Insights about commonalities in the human experience of loss are a boon for those wishing to create their own personal grief ritual. For the aimless bereaved individual fumbling in the dark, uncertain as to how they need to cope, the vast wisdom derived from an examination of cultural grief rituals can shine a light on viable options previously left in the dark and unconsidered. Those expressions of grief and mourning may guide the bereaved towards a more creative, restorative, and personally meaningful response to loss, but a slippery slope awaits.

Excavations into unfamiliar corners of the planet also expose our glaring ignorance regarding others' rituals and their underlying systems of meaning. Those who dig up cultural artifacts all too often fail to comprehend what they hold in their hands. Do we actually understand why Mexicans eat meals near the grave sites of their family members, or why cremation is preferred in Hindi cultures, or why some peoples routinely unearth the corpses of their dead years later only to bury them once more? Uncertainty abounds upon contemplating what the emotional component of loss and grief feels like for others, why the decisive moment of death is believed to occur when it does, or how different cultures manage to hold on to their relationship with the dead while simultaneously moving on. And so the problem of interpreting the meaning behind cultural grief rituals is twofold: We either fail to appreciate what is actually quite relatable or we risk minimizing important differences. Our discussion begins with the latter, what can be referred to as a problem of *assumed uniformity*.

Death itself is universal among humans. It is the great equalizer and is perhaps our most common denominator. But any kinship between two groups of people and how they experience death, grief, and mourning may very well end there. To fathom grief rituals and the mourning process beyond the familiarity of one's own culture proves to be quite the perplexing task, as we are forced to confront what is foreign and alien to our most deeply held assumptions about what grief looks and sounds like, as well as what it means to mourn a loss. Efforts to comprehend and appreciate the other are destined to fail if funneled through one's own preconceptions as a basis for interpretation. And the intrepid individual who is too eager to extract something relatable from the wisdom of another culture, something that may imbue the creation of a personal grief ritual with meaningful activity, risks taking in and embodying foreign behaviors they do not understand.

Anthropologists have long cautioned against the pitfalls of an outsider looking in and filtering interpretations of others' customs through their own ethnocentric, "etic" lens (this is in contrast to the "emic" understanding that comes from those within a culture). Clifford Geertz (1960) has gone so far as to posit that an outsider's interpretation of another culture's construction of meaning amounts to *nothing more than* one's own pre-existing construction of meaning. According to Metcalf and Huntington (1991), "the result is to mask the specialness of particular cultural configurations" (p. 11). Assumed uniformity collapses our ability to appreciate the unique bedrock of meaning that cultural grief rituals rest are built.

Consider the enormous differences in the degree to which noise is implemented amid mourning and the meaning behind the use of various sounds. The American funeral is unique in its insistence on quietude and softly spoken condolences. Whatever sounds that emerge from social relations among fellow mourners or from emotional expressions of grief are restrained and kept mum, and those familiar with this component of ritual expect others to grieve in a similarly dispassionate and sorrowful manner. But for many cultures, funerals are loud and rambunctious affairs. It is quite common for the bereaved to be rather boisterous and rowdy among one another. And this is not merely the result of permissive attitudes. Many communities actively encourage such behavior. What underlying meaning about grief and mourning spurs the bereaved to create such commotion at a funeral?

One answer is that noise in grief rituals delineates a transition from one moment of time to the next. Rodney Needham's (1967) aptly named paper "Percussion and Transition" declares that percussive instruments have tended to be associated with transitional rites of passage, such as weddings, births, and harvest festivals. Metcalf and Huntington (1991) expanded on this observation and applied it to the ways in which loud and *purposeful noisiness* in grief rituals demarcates the irreversible transition from life and presence in the past to death and absence moving forward.

Certain rituals create loud noise to denote the precise moment of death. The banging of drums or the ringing of bells proclaims that those who have been ill are now dead. Some, including natives of Hawaii, intentionally wail in order to announce that death has arrived (Green & Beckwith, 2009). The Berawan people from the island of Borneo – a large island in the Southeast Asian archipelago of Malay, which encompasses parts of Indonesia, Malaysia, and the nation of Brunei – ring a gong to announce death's arrival. And during funerals, the Berawan repeatedly deploy a large booming drum alongside the clanging gongs that can be heard for miles in all directions. Raucous games are played by men and women alike, and the great swell of cacophonous noise reaches its climax as shotguns are fired to signal that the corpse is being moved to the graveyard (Metcalf & Huntington, 1991).

Americans accustomed to quiet funerals would be incorrect to assume that an abundance of noise demonstrates an absence of mourning. Should the Berawan people act as interpreter of another culture's purposeful noisiness during grief rituals, they would be mistaken to assume it must be a declaration of death or a symbol of transition. Sound may be used instead to symbolize the raw emotions of grief and conjure up further emotional expression. Such is the case in the Jewish practice of *keriah*, in which the rending of garments worn at a funeral, often a black ribbon placed over the individual's heart, and the sound of fabric being torn express the wrenching pain of a loved one being violently ripped away (Levine, 1997). The noise created during keriah can also signify a transition in time or an acknowledgment of absence. Purposeful noise can also be sounded to evoke the presence of the deceased's spirit as well. In the Mexican holiday of Dia de los Meurtos, noise is used to wake the dead's spirit and coax them out so that the living may once more be present with their deceased loved ones (Carmichael & Sayer, 1992).

It seems that diverse communities of people around the world do not even agree upon a uniform color that represents death. Turner (1967) noted that, for many cultures in mourning, the various tones that predominate rituals and shows of grief correspond to one bodily association to death or another. Black, evoking images of rot and decay in the corpse, provides the backdrop to most cultures' funerals. Christians sometimes emphasize white as a symbol of the eternal life that death brings, whereas Australian Aborigines and the people of Borneo use white to symbolize "the pallor of death and the whiteness of bones" (Metcalf & Huntington, p. 63). And for mourners in Madagascar, red is the funerary hue of choice as blood represents a counterforce of life and vitality against the darkness of black and death. Conversely, red is strictly forbidden at Chinese funerals, as red traditionally designates happiness. Furthermore, it is believed that the deceased should not be dressed in red lest he or she transform into a ghost. White typically symbolizes death in Chinese culture.

Avoiding the low-hanging fruit of *assumed uniformity* is a satisfactory starting point in any effort to grasp the true meaning behind another culture's grief rituals. It is always beneficial to put aside one's own framework and maintain an open mind while inquiring into the other's potentially different experience of loss, grief, and mourning. But alas, an entirely separate challenge awaits. That which is unfamiliar at first glance is quickly cast aside as something eternally unknowable. We may even truncate our curiosity and deem the other to be engaged in nonsensical practices that hinder the mourning process and warrant no further consideration. Tempting as it may be to conclude that disparate peoples are so couched in idiosyncratic systems of meaning so radically alien to each other that they will never understand one another, the human experience of loss does bind us together in remarkable ways. Behind the veil of seemingly strange and bizarre rituals often lies something more recognizable than we had presumed, some aspect of ourselves embedded within another's behavior. The second impediment to our efforts to understand the meaning behind grief rituals is the tendency to *sensationalize the cultural other.*

Outside observations of other cultures' customary reactions to loss carry the potential to incite confusion, shock, bewilderment, or disgust. The dead may be artificially preserved or exposed to the elements of nature. Corpses are buried, burned, or consumed by bereaved survivors. Behaviors within grief rituals can be highly expressive or restrained. Funerals and prescribed mourning practices either isolate the bereaved from one another or encourage intimate interaction, some including raucous festivities, unabashed sexuality, and outpourings of joy, while others are marked by weeping, shows of sorrow, even self-injury.

Take, for instance, the following example of a particularly peculiar series of grief rituals. Upon receiving news of a loved one's death, a community of family and friends will huddle together and gaze at the deceased's corpse for an entire day. Every individual takes their turn approaching the dead as it lies in a supine position. In what appears to be a compulsory act, they walk slowly up to the corpse and comment on, of all things, the deceased's appearance. And the comments are invariably positive. The corpse is said to look "good" or "comfortable." An outside observer would notice the uncanny manner in which every bereaved individual conducts themselves. The range of emotion on display is limited to flat, solemn facial expressions. There is no unbridled wailing, no palpable shows of anger, nor are there any expressions of joy. The mood in the air is predictably and undeniably serious. A tear or two may be shed, but the horde of mourners grieves in an undifferentiated mass of quietude and restraint. Nor is there any noteworthy movement; in this culture, the bereaved stand still and talk politely with one another.

When the time comes to bury the dead, often the day after the initial viewing, the corpse is dressed in full attire not unlike what they would have worn while alive. The body is placed in an egregiously expensive wooden box, the insides of which are made to resemble comfortable bedding. Finally, the box is shut close and buried deep beneath the ground, forever out of sight to those who might wish to revisit their loved ones to mourn. The bereaved are left with few options moving forward other than to awkwardly return to the burial spot and once again sit immobile or stand still, gazing at the location of their loved one's final resting spot.

Many readers will have undoubtedly come to recognize this peculiar set of grief rituals as nothing more than the all-too-familiar American funeral. For those raised to be acquainted with these practices, there is nothing strange or curious about an open-casket funeral, during which stony-faced mourners stare at a fully dressed corpse and stand still until it is time to lower the casket into a burial plot. But any culture looking at another's customs from the outside will be inclined to see them as exotic, even absurd! Those who are unfamiliar with a typical American funeral would be left to ponder a host of oddities: Why is emotional expression so restrained? And why is there no opportunity to express any sustained feelings of joy or anger? Why is the deceased dressed as if they were still alive and the body made to look as if it were not decaying? And furthermore, why is the body interred underground . . . and for a fee at that?

This intentionally dramatic description of a typical American funeral is an exercise meant to evoke surprise where there had been familiarity, to see how that which is usually brushed aside as undeserving of a closer look is, in actuality, rather intriguing despite how accustomed one may be with it. Marcus and Fischer (1986) refer to this technique as *defamiliarization by cross-cultural juxtaposition*, a helpful way to raise conscious awareness of differences between cultures by uncovering all that is surreal and uncanny in the familiar. Those practices enacted close to home may very well be just as curious as those abroad, and this realization hopefully begins to allay unduly negative reactions to the cultural other. Differing practices are to be studied and considered with genuine respect and awe rather than be sensationalized or, even worse, dismissed.

Different cultures' grief rituals undoubtedly seem strange from afar, but those who scrutinize what they do not understand are left scratching their heads upon realizing that their distant neighbors are doing just fine. The cultural other continues to grieve and adapt to life. And while the success of one might be taken to imply that alternative prescriptions for mourning are ill-advised, myriad approaches all carry the potential to help their community mourn. Equipped with greater open-mindedness, perhaps we can then reserve judgment when contemplating, say, the reasons some grief rituals entail leaving the deceased's body outside to be consumed by animals, or the preference for cremation over interment in the ground, or of those cultures who opt to keep the corpse of their family members nearby well after death and interact with them during daily activities, or grief rituals that encourage joyful celebration and dancing, or of tribes in remote corners of the world that have found immense meaning in consuming the flesh of their deceased loved ones. Perhaps the quiet and somber expressions at American funerals, along with their compulsory viewing of and positive commentary on a fully dressed corpse lying in a bed, are no less bizarre.

"Assumed uniformity" and "sensationalizing the cultural other" amount to a two-pronged error in interpreting the function and meaning behind cultural grief rituals. Where the former leads us to conclude that our neighbors' practices are *more similar* to our own than they really are, the latter runs the risk of seeing our neighbors as unnecessarily *unknowable*. This seems contradictory. Either we can understand other cultures' behaviors or it is beyond the reach of our empathy. Such perils of dichotomous thinking leave both the curious layperson and the scholar at a standstill.

A dialectic synthesis of these two seemingly incompatible interpretations is in order. Disparate cultures are notably different from one another, and their uniqueness should be studied with curiosity and reverence; nonetheless, others' practices often attempt to facilitate similar functions of mourning – emotional expression, acceptance of the finality of death, an ongoing abstract connection to the dead, and forward movement after the loss – albeit in markedly different manners, in varying degrees, and with different conclusions about the course that mourning is to take. This is because *cultural grief rituals are tailored to the unique meaning structures and specific psychological needs of the community*. That these Wordenesque tasks are at the center of most cultures' practices is of little surprise. It is, however, a jolt to one's presuppositions to discover that disparate peoples hold radically different beliefs about *how* to facilitate these tasks of mourning. To further explore how the same tasks of mourning can be addressed in wildly divergent ways, we will now consider how different cultures produce different answers to the following questions: When does death occur? What does grief feel like?

When does death occur?: Liminality and rites of transition

At what precise moment is the deceased considered . . . dead? Surprisingly, there is no consensus about how to answer this question. Numerous beliefs abound about when the soul has been emancipated from its earthly ties, rendering the body no more than an empty vessel. Western medical traditions assert that the cessation of neuronal activity in the brain ushers in the decisive moment, at which point the doctor marks the precise time of death. But some are not so quick to declare that death has arrived, pointing to the days and weeks after the cessation of breath, when fingernails and hair continue to grow, suggesting that trace elements of life remain and that death is not so instantaneous. The Hindu practice of cremating the deceased on a funeral pyre holds that death has not taken place until the extreme heat causes the skull to split, one of many in a sequence of rites that occur days after the deceased has taken their final breath. And the deceased is not considered to be truly dead in many cultures until the body has completely decomposed, years after the mind and body have been immobilized; this particular belief has given rise to elaborate customs and rituals that embrace a slower and steadier process. Death, for many, is not a butcher knife that decisively cleaves off life from the bone!

The Tana Toraja of Indonesia live alongside the bodies of their deceased relatives for years (Budiman, 2013). As the deceased are not yet thought to be resolutely dead, family members are permitted to slowly come to terms with each loss in due time. Relatives who have ceased breathing are propped up in chairs in the home and spoken of as *the sleeping person* until the funeral begins, often years later. Children still play with their deceased grandparents. Mothers and fathers continue to care for their deceased children with portions of food and warm clothing. These practices may appear to do no more than perpetuate a fantasy that thwarts the necessity of relinquishing ties and accepting reality, but Torajans report that maintaining a relationship with the deceased provides emotional comfort and eases the prolonged process of mourning.

As we will soon see, a host of cultures engage in similar mourning practices and rituals which throw a wrench into the works of any presupposition about when the moment of death occurs. If death is not considered to be an instantaneous event upon the cessation of biological life, how do the bereaved determine when death has finally arrived? And what is to be made of the ongoing relationship with the deceased in the interim? In order to better understand these practices and begin answering such confounding questions, we must turn to the anthropological concept of *liminality*.

A fifteen-year-old Mexican girl celebrates her quinceañera and, in doing so, marks the transition from girlhood to womanhood. Two individuals who wish to spend their lives intimately bound together participate in a wedding ceremony, abandoning their single status to become married. Years of study in a university commence with a graduation ceremony, and with the turning of the cap's tassel from right to left, the student transforms into a graduate.

The transitional sequence in each rite described above seems to be rather straightforward: distance oneself from the previous status – girlhood, being single, student – and adopt a new status – womanhood, married, graduate – upon completion of the rite. But in Arnold van Gennep's (1960) seminal work *The Rites of Passage*, he noted that rites of passage are more complex than a binary transition from one status to another; instead, they are organized around a tripartite sequence with a crucial middle phase. There is an initial period of separation from one status, followed by *a transitional period*, and then concluding with reincorporation into a new status. This intermediary phase came to be known as *liminality*, which denotes the disorienting and ambiguous quality of having relinquished one status without having yet fully adopted the new. The fourteen-year-old prepares for her quinceañera, and although she may no longer feel like such a little girl, nor does she feel like a woman just yet. The couple that has committed themselves to marriage and a life in union enters an awkward phase of being engaged, where nothing has changed about their lives together and yet the relationship does not feel quite the same as before even as they orient themselves to what they will become. The college student completes his or her final class, abandons the status of student, and attends a graduation ceremony, during which the ambiguity of what comes next in life weighs heavy. Individuals within the liminal stage of a rite of passage stand at the threshold between their previous identity or role in the community and their eventual destination, neither here nor there.

Van Gennep observed that the majority of ceremonies and rituals are less oriented towards rites of separation or reincorporation and more towards complex and prolonged *rites of transition*. Robert Hertz (1960) and Victor Turner (1969) extended this observation and applied it to the ubiquity of rites of transition within funeral ceremonies and various death rituals. For instance, in Robert Hertz's classic study of secondary burials, he discovered that Berawan people of Borneo reserve a period of time for an intermediary experience of loss and mourning. Surviving family and community members relinquish their ties ever so gradually, for while the Berawan conceive of the deceased as no longer living, they are not considered dead just yet. The bereaved stand at the threshold of experiencing loss and absence as absolute. This liminal phase persists until the remains of the corpse, having been stored in a longhouse or on a simple platform within a graveyard, are completely decomposed, a process that often takes years. The Berawan mark the end of mourning with an elaborate gathering and feast. The deceased's remains are then prepared for their more conclusive entombment within a coffin and ultimately relocated to their final resting spot in a nearby mausoleum (Metcalf, 1976).

The Malagasy people of Madagascar practice a rather-infamous ritual called famadihana, or the *turning of the bones*. Once every five to seven years, families invite anywhere from a few dozen to several hundred guests to join them at their ancestral crypt, where the bodies of the dead are exhumed, wrapped in fresh silk shrouds, and sprayed with wine or perfume. Guests are fed indulgent meals, and musicians are hired to play music, while family members dance with the corpses around the tomb. It is a lively and joyous celebration. Living relatives relay family news to the deceased, request their blessings, and ask the deceased for any wisdom they can impart onto the ritual's guests. Famadihana is also a time to rekindle old memories and share stories of the dead with one another. Once the festivities have ended, the deceased are returned to their crypt once more (Holloway, 2014).

Akin to the Japanese practice of ancestor worship and their belief in a permeable boundary between life and death, the Malagasy believe that the deceased's spirit can pass back and forth between these worlds. This is an unfortunate fate for all if the deceased remain in limbo, forever haunting the living and never arriving at their final destination. Effectively stuck in between worlds of the living and the dead, the deceased are still considered to be alive until the appropriate number of famadihana rituals has been carried out. The living are responsible for carrying out this ritual every five to seven years until it is clear that the body has completely decomposed, thus facilitating a definitive passage into the world of the ancestors (Holloway, 2014).

Similar practices have been discovered in societies spanning from the Berawan people of Indonesia to the Choctaw Native Americans of Oklahoma (only until the early nineteenth century) to the ancient Zoroastrians of Iran and the *Towers of Silence* they once relied upon while patiently waiting for the body of the deceased to be ready for a final burial (Kerrigan, 2017). These rituals draw attention to the variety of perspectives regarding the temporal nature of death as well as the appropriate length of time required in order to transition through mourning.

Cultural anthropologist Victor Turner (1967) built upon van Gennep's work on liminality and advanced Hertz's observations on secondary burial, offering ingenious insights into the liminal phase of any given culture's grief rituals and what they reveal about how a collection of people conceptualizes death. Turner argued that *the fate of the body represents how a society conceives of the soul's fate.* And for many, beliefs about death and the soul go beyond a simple binary of the deceased having once been alive and then being dead; their beliefs and practices hinge upon a three-part sequence marked by the crucial intermediary of liminality: alive . . . dying . . . dead.

Let us once again consider the liminal phase of mourning as it relates to those who practice secondary burial. The decaying and putrid body remains in a prolonged process of change that moves ever closer to death. Although the deceased has separated from the world of the living, he or she has not yet arrived in the world of the dead, be it the land of ancestors, heaven, or some other variation of an afterlife. The deceased remain homeless in effect and are thought to be capable of inflicting dread and hostility towards the living until only dry, imperishable bones remain. Only at this point has the soul migrated to and been incorporated into the afterlife, effectively ending the liminal phase of transition.

Turner's insight into secondary burials complements Metcalf and Huntington's central thesis that studying the symbolic attributes assigned to the dead offers insight into a culture's view of death. The Berawan of Borneo are one of many peoples who harbor fear of the corpse, but their dread is not a matter of corporeal disgust or aversion to decay itself. It is believed that time must destroy the body of the deceased before the soul can transcend. Mourners wait patiently, always in fear of the deceased's spiritual essence remaining present and inflicting harm before it has properly transformed and transitioned. The eventual act of secondary burial serves to confirm that the body has decomposed in full and that the spirit can advance towards its final destination, thus unburdening the bereaved. For the sake of mourning, the dissolution and rotting of the body carry highly positive connotations.

In contrast, the American funeral places a great premium on ensuring that the dead look dignified in nice clothing and cozy within their bedded coffin before being buried forever out of sight. This suggests that the primary concerns in death, as in American life, are whether or not the soul will have material comforts and find ease in the afterlife. Efforts to preserve the appearance of life and vibrancy in the corpse make it clear that the American view of death and decay is that it is by no means eagerly awaited but that it is to be feared and turned away from. Furthermore, by comparison to the lengthy liminal phase of secondary burial, the swift progression from death to burial parallels the American view that grief and mourning are to be processed and moved beyond at breakneck speed. Conversely, for those cultures that practice secondary burial, the dead's slow decay and persistent ability to haunt the living lays bare their belief that death, as well as the proper course of mourning, is a prolonged process.

Turner also noticed that many cultures see the rotting body and the dissolution of its form as *an important metaphor for both the deceased and the bereaved.* Just as there is thought to be a liminal phase in which the deceased is slowly separating from this world and transitioning into the next, so too is the community of mourners steadily parting with physical attachment to loved ones and readying themselves for a new life without the dead, however incrementally. This observation provides a moving analogy of what mourning entails regardless of one's beliefs about when death occurs: We all aim to strike the correct balance between holding on while simultaneously letting go in due time.

However slow or fast the liminal phase unfolds, those in mourning must eventually transition out of a state of acute mourning and back into life with resumed purpose and vibrancy. This is why many cultures' rites of separation eventually find their way towards efforts to reincorporate the bereaved back into life. On the Andaman Islands, a territory of India just southwest of Myanmar, the Andamanese weep while embracing the deceased's corpse. Mourners in such an affective state are considered to be temporarily enveloped within the world of the dead. But as shows of sorrow and persistent attachment to the deceased finally recede, mourners are reunited with their community, effectively pulled back into the world of the living, albeit a world marked by a notable absence (Radcliffe-Brown, 1964).

Seeing as how the pursuit of new life after a loss is of utmost importance, it is not surprising to find that the liminal phase of death rituals is often bursting at the seams with sexual energy. It is quite common for funerals to morph into rowdy affairs filled with energetic dancing, demonstrations of sexual prowess, and unabashed flirtations. An inseparable pair, death and life are woven together; the vitality of sexual symbolism serves as a counterbalance to the cold and breathless sterility of death. Death rites and rituals are replete with paradoxical symbols of rebirth in hopes that the dead will be released from one world and be born, as it were, into the world of their ancestors.

The Nyakyusa people of Tanzania and Malawi mourn death and celebrate life in lockstep. The Nyakyusa funeral is a festive event in which dancing and flirtation are encouraged. The men gyrate to the sounds of drumming to honor the dead with shows of virility and courage on their behalf. By contrast, the females act as the designated *owners of death*, whose persistent wailing while indoors with the corpse compartmentalizes the fearful trembling associated with grief. As the drumming swells to an ever-louder climax, dancing grows more and more energetic, often infused with strong elements of sexuality. Nyakyusa culture fears the afterworld and that the lingering spirit of the deceased will bring great misfortune to its people. The cacophony of drumming and the frenetic energy of dancing aim to drive away the spirit (Wilson, 1939).

The Bara people of Madagascar enact their own variation of secondary burial with a heavy dose of sexual symbolism. In preparation for reburial, the coffin is placed within the *house of many tears* and is guarded by young women. The men of the village, intent on retrieving the coffin, storm into the house and steal away with the dead, at which point the young women are to give chase and make a show of struggle as they attempt to wrest the coffin back to the village. Metcalf and Huntington (1991) noted how this behavior closely resembles a game of tug-of-war. However, the premeditated struggle is doomed to fail. Its crucial moment comes when the young women run ahead and create a barrier, which the men must penetrate with the coffin en route to the tomb that will be the deceased's final resting spot and the beginning of their new journey.

Metcalf and Huntington (1991) have observed the ubiquity of this phenomenon, saying, "Some association of sex with death occurs in nearly every culture in the world" (p. 25). Metaphors of death and rebirth often accompany one another. Like a New Year's Eve party attended by personifications of both the specter of death and a newborn baby standing side by side as the last seconds of the year tick away, the old is relinquished while ushering in the new. And just as death rituals are charged with elements of sexuality and rebirth that aid in the deceased's final transition, so too does the bereaved benefit from assertions of their own vitality and forward movement amid the malaise of grief. From the ashes of prolonged liminality emerge rituals of reincorporation that leave death behind in pursuit of fresh life. The bereaved survivor of death must also be reborn.

Liminality is embedded into even the most mundane moments of our daily routines, our jobs, and our relationships. An early-morning shower finds you no longer asleep but not yet quite awake. As you step into your car on the way to work, you still remain tethered to your home for a moment yet simultaneously in transit to a location at which you have not yet arrived. And the surreal experience of being at an airport finds one neither here nor there. Even the conversations we hold with one another regularly begin with small talk that pulls us out of loneliness while still leaving us yearning for something that will hopefully come to feel like the deep connection for which we yearn.

However gradually we transition from one state of consciousness to another, or travel from one location to the next, or slowly edge our way into intimacy, it is imperative that we eventually step beyond such ambiguous middle ground and reach a destination. Some spaces, both literal and figurative, are not meant to be occupied indefinitely. Standing inert in the shower all morning neglects the clock. Lingering in a parking lot for too long evokes an uncanny sense of inertia and unease, as if one should be en route towards their next location. The blissful rapture of sex grows awkward and frustrating if its desired conclusion is delayed or uncertain. The bereaved must venture through mourning and eventually arrive at a satisfactory distance from the initial shock of separation and sorrow.

Grief rituals chart a course through the liminal phase of mourning. The meaningful behaviors and symbolic gestures prescribed by any given culture beckon the bereaved away from what was, guides them through the tangled thicket of grief, and ultimately leads them to what lies ahead. The bereaved, often lost in the dark without ritual to navigate them through, are eager to follow whatever path their culture lays out. And in response to the question of "When does death occur?" the bereaved will act in accordance with however their culture answers, be it the immediacy of death as the absence of neurological activity or the prolonged liminality of waiting for corporeal decay. But some individuals are pulled to defect from the communal path and find their own stride. Just as one culture struggles to understand why an unfamiliar group of people moves through mourning as fast or as slow as they do, *the individual may be at odds with the pace at which his or her own culture tells them to separate from and relinquish their bonds.*

What does loss feel like?: The internal experience of grief and its ritualized exhibition

Death is the only constant. Universal in its reach, our eventual demise binds us all together more intimately than anything else. And so it is tempting to presume that we are bound further by a common reaction *to* death; grief, we assume, is akin to a ubiquitous wince of pain upon burning one's finger. Nonetheless, the internal and subjective experience of grief is far from uniform. There is, in fact, a vast chasm between the ways in which many cultures express the emotional component of mourning differently from another. A kaleidoscopic array of feelings may emerge among one group that another would never exhibit. Some cry sorrowful tears where others tremble in fear, exude anger, or revel in joy.

But any effort to answer the question of "What does grief feel like?" runs up against a much more perplexing conundrum: *What is the relationship between the internal experience of grief and the external display of such?* Anthropologists have long wondered if grief rituals open a pathway for the outward expression of emotions that had already been felt within or if they are mere exhibitions designed to cull out predetermined responses which culture deems appropriate. It is surprisingly difficult to ascertain which precedes the other, a causality dilemma of "the chicken or the egg" proportions.

Grief rituals may very well play a role in facilitating genuine emotional expression. They regularly incorporate meaningful symbols and behavioral gestures to coax out internal states of grief believed to have arisen naturally in the bereaved. For instance, funeral ceremonies around the world encourage participants to alter standard grooming practices as a meaningful indication of their internal state. Hindus regularly shave their heads as an expression of grief, a symbolic representation of death having wrested away an important relationship and, in turn, a part of the self now felt to be missing (Laungani, 1997). Women in Australian Aboriginal culture also cut their hair or engage in self-harming behaviors as ritualized outlets for conveying feelings of pain amid their mourning (Farrelly & Francis, 2009). Other cultures intentionally neglect hygiene and grooming in a show of outward dishevelment to match the internal state of chaos and disorganization that has fallen upon the bereaved. Should deep feelings of anguish spring up, a ritual like the rending of cloth in *keriah* is created to draw it out.

Indeed, we are inclined to think of grief rituals as facilitating a path towards catharsis for something that had been otherwise pent up. Metcalf and Huntington (1991) wrote, "The potentiality of death to release the most powerful emotions in the survivors is so obvious that it is often assumed to explain the rites that follow" (p. 2). And yet a survey of various cultures' customs surrounding death gives ample reason to claim the inverse: *Enactment of ritual precedes the felt experience of emotion*. From this perspective, the behavioral elements of grief rituals are not necessarily drawing out genuine emotions that originated within the bereaved and had already been *felt*. Whatever emotions are on display during grief rituals – sorrow, fear, joy, or anger – may represent an assigned performance for the bereaved to act out in compliance with the feeling state-ordained in advance per cultural beliefs and values. The internal experience of grief and outward expression of such are not necessarily one and the same.

It may be that the drive to feel connected to fellow mourners shapes the design of grief rituals more than the need to express what arises from within. Sociologist Emile Durkheim (1965) posited that the primary purpose of ritual is to bind members of a community together and ensure solidarity through participation in mutually meaningful activities. Functional anthropologists, such as Robert Hertz (1960) and Alfred Radcliffe-Brown (1964), agree that the most essential and beneficial function of participation in any ritual is that they instill feelings of group cohesion and connectedness. And in the case of grief rituals, it is the collective experience of death, grief, and mourning which must be affirmed.

To this end, a culture's rituals revolve around a system of sacred symbols set apart from the mundane doldrums of life and revered as inherently meaningful to its participants. A wooden cross in Christian funerals, smoke undulating from an incense stick during Dia de los Muertos, or the lighting of a yahrzeit candle during the Jewish ritual of sitting shiva provides a focal point around which all gather to share a collective experience of emotion, including the affective component of what loss and grief feel like. The bereaved participate in the sacred and interact with its symbols, evoking what Durkheim called *effervescence*, a collective welling up of intense emotions. In grief rituals, the experience of feeling potent emotions in unison with one another, be it exaltation or listless sorrow, sparks a powerful bond and strengthens group cohesion, thus motivating a return to the community that ensures ongoing solidarity.

Durkheim's theory argues that the social structure of ritual *creates* the sentiment and that the ritual's purpose is to make the socially prescribed sentiments *become* genuinely felt and amplified through participation. This astute observation complements one of many intriguing theories in psychology on the subjective experience of emotion. The James-Lange theory of emotion has long asserted that external stimuli create physiological responses in the body which are then interpreted as emotional reactions (Lange, 1912). A racing heart rate and sweaty palms are subsequently experienced as anxiety. Clenched jaws and a hot feeling in the neck provoke the interpretation that one must be feeling angry. When participating in grief rituals, the emotional experience of a loss is born in the external enactment of rites and through interaction with sacred symbols.

Rational-choice theories argue that rituals are ubiquitous features of social life because they create *common knowledge* that help a community of individuals coordinate their actions with increased efficiency. Indeed, Birx (2006) has observed that rituals quite simply serve to clarify how mourners in the community are to behave while in mourning. Amid the backdrop of chaos and disorder that ensue after loss, common cultural knowledge about how to grieve affords the bereaved a semblance of predictability and familiar structure. Each bereaved individual can orient his or her emotional expression of grief towards what can be expected from the group, and in seeing their affect mirrored back to them, the bereaved find reassurance and validation of their feelings (Chwe, 2001). Participants within a ritual may fail to realize that the emotional experience is determined in advance and artificially coaxed out for the sake of efficiency. Nonetheless, this positive feedback loop binds people together in times of distress and great uncertainty.

Symbols clearly play a role in the expression of emotion during grief rituals, but here, too, the relationship between the external symbol and the internal emotion remains uncertain. Perhaps the rending of cloth performed during keriah is not so much a purge of distress as it is a socially sanctioned exhibition of the kind and quantity of pain determined to be appropriate after a loss. Cutting one's hair as a gesture of mourning may be no more than an obligatory show of collective distress that obscures the true and unfeigned emotional reaction to loss that resides within each individual mourner.

Many cultures' rituals are flexible and allow some room for the errant individual's emotions to burst forth and break from the script. A spontaneous cry of grief may disrupt an otherwise-quiet event. While delivering a eulogy, the bereaved might diverge from his solemn tone and crack a light-hearted joke or shake his hands in anger before returning to his somber stance at the pulpit. While the structure of certain rituals tolerates variability and is organized around mere suggestions for how the majority are to emote, the manifestation of a particular emotion is compulsory in many cultures' customs. Furthermore, demonstration of grief is often scripted in rigid sequences that emerge and screech to a halt for all mourners at precise, predetermined moments.

Radcliffe-Brown (1964) studied the Andaman Islanders' mourning customs and how a host of mandatory expressions of sorrow serves to "affirm the existence of a social bond between two or more persons" (pg. 240). Custom dictated that such emotional display was expected among every member of the community regardless of whether or not the sentiment is actually felt. Within certain Arab sects, bereaved family members are compelled to cry loudly in great shows of anguish (Parkes, 1997). And in Hawaiian culture, it is customary after cleaning and dressing the body of the deceased to intentionally broadcast loud bursts of wailing as a signal for family and community to pour into the home of the bereaved (Green & Beckwith, 2009). The funeral rituals of native Australian Aborigines reveal an obligatory exhibition of emotion in which the pain of mourning, or *sorry business*, is signaled by an outpouring of piercing cries and a zenith of exasperated pain and anger that may only gain its fullest expression by means of self-inflicted *sorry cuts* thought to bring about a release of pain through bloodletting (Farrelly & Francis, 2009). Individuals participating in these customs and rituals may very well be expressing an internal state of grief they genuinely feel, but many are simply conveying what their culture expects of them.

Others' customs strictly *forbid* the expression of certain emotions. The Bara of Madagascar prohibit crying during preparations for burial, and not far away, the Malagasy of Madagascar discourage tears during their famadihana ceremonies, particularly during moments when the bodies are exhumed and again when they are interred once more into the ground (Metcalf & Huntington, 1991). Buddhists, preferring a calm emotional response at the bedside of the dying, may decide to exclude distressed family members from being nearby (Parkes, 1997).

Many theories about the emotional expression of grief hold the cynical view that rituals are bent on squashing the mundane concerns of the individual, what Durkheim referred to as the *profane*, in deference to the sacred interests of the group. Bloch and Parry (1982) saw ritual as a mere source of social control that shapes emotional responses for its participants so as to deter individual expression. Kottak (2002) discussed one form of social control he called *leveling mechanisms*, those customs or social actions that aim to reduce differences between individuals and bring everyone in line with communal norms.

Nonetheless, individuals continually resonate with an array of feelings pertaining to their own personal experience of loss and mourning. This is particularly apparent in moments when the individual's affective display fails to meet cultural expectations and is met with disapproval. As much as culture often plays the role of puppet master, dictating its members' movements while in mourning, it does not pull all the strings. The individual maintains a modicum of autonomy over how they express the internal state of their grief. But bereaved individuals within a community stand to experience great frustration when culturally approved grief rituals do not draw out what begs for catharsis or explicitly blockade what only begins to emerge.

A brief digression on the absurdities of the American funeral

The manner in which a society conceptualizes and deals with death proves to be strongly associated with its core values about life. Each culture exhibits markedly different beliefs about the soul, the meaning of dreams that involve the dead, etiquette regarding what is worn while mourning, and one's communal obligations when it is time to participate in grief rituals (Rosenblatt, 1997). The traditional American funeral is not without its own brand of rites that showcase its culture's central ethos regarding life, death, and the emotional experience of mourning. Its hallmarks are threefold: embalming the corpse, gathering to view the body lying in a casket, and subsequent disposal by burial. Metcalf and Huntington (1991) proposed two factors – one of a psychological basis, and another economic – that elucidate the driving forces of meaning behind this curious triumvirate.

The historical origins of the American funeral can be traced back quite clearly to the midnineteenth century. In *Inventing the American Way of Death, 1830–1920*, James Farrell (1980) noted that the evolution of customs and rituals surrounding death in the United States took their most decisive turn as institutions that manage the dead, funeral parlors most notably, rose to prominence. Embalming techniques, which had been under development since the early nineteenth century, gained widespread use during the American Civil War as an efficient way to ship bodies of deceased soldiers long distances home, stave off decay in transit, and allow ample time for mourners to return home to attend a wake. Simultaneously, funeral directors usurped the once ever-present role of the church in matters of death and mourning. Whereas Jewish and Roman Catholic practices had discouraged open-casket viewings, funeral directors began putting their newly developed techniques and handiwork on display for the bereaved to behold. A viewing of the preserved corpse soon became one of the most defining aspects of the American funeral.

Emerging philosophical and scientific currents of the nineteenth century also played a role in chiseling away the traditional relationship between life and death. The ascension of scientific naturalism, with its Darwinian assertions that human death is a mere biological event no more significant than a grape withering on the vine, stripped mortality of its mystery and awe. Many came to believe that life no longer needed to be spent contemplating one's eventual place in the afterlife. And increasingly liberal attitudes about religion relieved people from the looming specter of hell and punishment. With life less oriented towards making a case for the providence of God after death, the individual was granted greater jurisdiction over his or her days, even if they be spent in fear and denial of our eventual quietus.

This sea change cultivated a culture in which the American psyche is now plagued by profound avoidance and fear of death. With increased institutionalization, bereaved family members were unburdened of the messy work of being in contact with the dying and the dead. Americans were permitted to avoid confrontations with mortality and repress contemplation of such, albeit at the expense of rendering death unthinkable and unspeakable. This is perhaps most evident in the cold and austere hospital rooms of terminally ill patients, where the blunt reality of inevitable death is seldom discussed, and the improbable hope of a miraculous recovery is clung to until the absolute final moments of life when the EKG heart monitor goes flatline.

With the ascent of funeral directors and their management of the body, most Americans find themselves immersed within a culture so averse to the deceased's body and beset with corporeal fear that they are deprived of any opportunity for hands-on involvement or active participation in meaningful rituals. The entire experience of mourning in America is characterized by passivity. The bereaved is cast into an increasingly uninvolved role.

Unlike those cultures who are in regular contact with the body after death, the corpse is immediately whisked away from the hospital to a funeral parlor and handled by professionals. The family may be expected to play no more significant role than to select the outfit in which the dead will be buried. Embalming and open-casket viewings perpetuate a large-scale pattern of the bereaved avoiding confrontation with decay and ultimate putrescence. Efforts are made to prepare, package, and present the corpse as a beautiful specimen to be gazed upon. Indeed, the bereaved do no more than look at their loved ones before letting go; they partake in an illusion that time has been frozen in place, an absurd and appalling denial of temporality. Even the symbolism of the dead lying peacefully in a casket made to look like a bed highlights a central theme of subdued acquiescence, a quiet whimper devoid of adequate protest. Custom dictates that the mourner is to comment with reticence on how the corpse looks good and how the dead appear to be peacefully at rest. And the burial proves to be of little meaning as well. The bereaved individual's presence at the grave site is equally unavailing, as it is commonplace to only stay briefly and then leave to let the professionals complete the interment. The mourner's hands remain a bit too clean.

If the American funeral looks like fear, its rituals smell like money. So said Jessica Mitford (1963) in her well-known exposé of the American funeral industry, *The American Way of Death*. Mitford pulled no punches in her scathing critique of a culture whose ethos and management of death lay bare its central values of materialism and ruthless commercialism. With the church and synagogue having abdicated many important aspects of managing death and mourning, funeral directors injected their own ethos into American death rites. It was Mitford's charge that the funeral industry is compromised by their association with the National Funeral Directors Association, who use political power to oppose cremation and profit from exploiting emotionally vulnerable clientele into buying expensive coffins and cemetery plots. The American mourner is rendered passive in most funerary functions, but they remain directly involved in a cornerstone of their culture: the purchasing of superfluous goods and services.

A well-known painting entitled *George Washington on His Deathbed* depicts what has largely disappeared from the culture's handling of death over the past two centuries. The former president is pictured lying in bed at home. It is a warm setting, with carpeted floors, ample pillows to support his head, and soft blankets of emerald green and an orange-tinted red. He is surrounded by family and friends looking on with sorrowful expressions, some of whom are hovering nearby in direct eye contact with their dying friend. Mr. Washington appears cognizant and engaged in his own death, as if courageously readying himself to say goodbye to his loved ones. This deathbed scene, which once provided so many individuals with an opportunity to confront death and grief head-on, is largely unrecognizable today.

So what values do American grief rituals *now* promulgate about the role of emotional expression in mourning? It seems that death and subsequent grief are to be feared and sidestepped. Emotions are to be restrained at the American funeral sparring the periodic venting of muted sadness. And what, according to American belief systems, do their rituals suggest about when death is thought to occur? A cultural emphasis on scientific naturalism and a deep-rooted aversion to the dead body spur on quick pronouncement of biological death. This is followed by a speedy interment and burial far beneath the surface, where the body remains forever out of sight, unable to disturb the living in their pursuit of life, liberty, and happiness.

There is reason to be hopeful that fear and avoidance of death have begun to loosen their grip on the American psyche. Mitford's critical analysis of the American funeral, Elizabeth Kubler-Ross's (1969) well-known research into the terminally ill patient's experience of dying, and Ernest Becker's (1973) anthropological study of profound unconscious denial of death heralded a *death awareness movement* that brought death out of the closet and revived public discourse about our curious relationship to mortality. Americans are not quite as mum on the topic as they once were, and recent trends suggest that the general public is growing less squeamish about alternative methods of disposing the body, including cremation. Nonetheless, Americans' peculiar practices have remained remarkably stable and intact.

It is far too easy to criticize American culture and what its rituals convey about their uneasy relationship with death, but an emphasis on contained emotional expression and a quick confirmation of life's finality is not without its benefits. For all we know, American values of industriousness, discovery, and innovation may be indebted, in part, to the fact that thoughts of mortality are repressed throughout much of daily life. And the majority of its citizens – estimates range from 80 to 90 percent – seem to proceed through the mourning process devoid of significant complications (Bonanno, 2004). Brief participation in funerary rites along with a touch of sorrow may very well suffice for the majority of American individuals.

And let us make no mistake about it: Other cultures' beliefs and grief rituals are wrought with their own serious flaws. As previously discussed, custom often *insists* upon embodying intense emotions the individual may not feel after a loss, and certain rituals *demand* that the bereaved remain in prolonged states of mourning beyond whatever amount of time the individual may truly need. In some corners of the world, women are barred from experiencing joy or intimacy. Others still justify cannibalism or ongoing contact with the corpse, which exposes the community to various pathogens. These rituals may be meaningful to those who practice them, but social pressure to remain in a state of inauthentic distress is oppressive, and proximity to decaying flesh, or the consumption of it, continues to give rise to widespread disease and health crises across entire communities, most noteworthy of which was a recent resurgence of the bubonic plague in Madagascar as the living mingled with the putrefied corpses of their loved ones. In those instances when tradition begins to fail more than whom they assist, a process of dissolution ensues, and in its vacuum awaits an opportunity for the creation of new grief rituals.

A square peg in a round hole: How rituals fail

Cultural grief rituals persist as long as participation satiates the societal and psychological needs of its members and achieves the crucial functions needed in order to facilitate mourning. The Berawan's secondary burials make certain that the reality of loss is actualized in due time, and the customs of those in the Sanyuan Village of China provide the soon-to-be bereaved an opportunity to say goodbye. Rending of cloth in the Jewish tradition of keriah and the Hawaiians' insistence on wailing guarantee that the emotional pains of separation will be wrung out. The Bara and Nyakyusa incorporation of dance and flirtation in their rituals ensures that both the deceased and the bereaved alike will be propelled towards a new and vital plane of existence after death. The Mexican tradition of Dia de los Muertos helps cultivate and maintain an ongoing meaningful relationship with the deceased.

But rituals do not always scratch what itches. Metcalf and Huntington (1991) suggest that the performance of death rituals and the psychological process of grieving might only intersect partially, saying, "it may be that ritual sometimes aids the process, but it could as easily be no help at all, or even an extra burden to bear" (pg. 5). Under what conditions do rituals fail to facilitate mourning and, instead, create discontent within those who participate? Furthermore, what happens when the underlying meaning and structures of tradition buckle under the pressures of frustration and begin to crumble?

We recall that numerous cultural anthropologists have suggested that funeral rituals are expressions of a society's cohesion and serve to recreate and reaffirm the sentiments that a community depends on in order to bolster solidarity. Durkheim (1965), as fervent a champion of this notion as anyone, was also willing to address inherent tensions between the collective group and each individual within it. Participation in rituals may very well stave off isolation, but it often does so at the expense of alienating the individual from his or her autonomy and the pursuit of authentic personal meaning about a loss. Durkheim expressed concern that members of a community, for the sake of social solidarity, will repress what feels genuine and place moral pressure on themselves to alter their behavior to be in harmony with the collective and its venerated symbols. The individual loses himself. He becomes swallowed up in identification with an undifferentiated mass of thoughts and feelings belonging to the group; the ritual fails to evoke genuine sadness or anger or joy. The individual finds themselves in rigid lockstep with others' actions instead of following their intuition. Thus, the ritual fails to provide an opportunity for meaningful acts of mourning.

Neo-Durkheimian theorists insist that a theory of rituals must specify circumstances under which rituals fail to produce collective emotions as they once did and how its focus gets redirected to the creation of new sacred objects. Giesen (2006) voiced concern that rituals can ironically *inhibit* the very spontaneous emotional catharsis they aim to facilitate. Collins (2004) added that rituals often produce "little or no feeling of group solidarity; no sense of one's identity affirmed or changed; no respect for the group's symbols; no heightened emotional energy" (p. 51). But where Giesen signals an alarm that participation in rituals simply does not guarantee social order and cohesiveness, Collins rings the bell louder, observing how formal rituals can produce dissonant emotions and discord among its participants, ironically weakening social relations in the process and giving way to the decay of rituals that had intended to bind a community together.

Furthermore, rituals can take on a quality of *stale ceremonialism* as they are passed down from one generation to the next (Calhoun & Gerteis, 2012). Those sequences of behavior that arose organically out of a different context and system of meaning, which once produced social solidarity and made manifest the emotions of grief, feel inappropriately imported from another time; stale ceremonialism is a foreboding black box weathered by too much time. And participation in anachronistic rituals comes to feel awkwardly imposed rather than creating the illusion of a spontaneous fit of collective grief. Compulsive incantations steeped in tired tradition distract from what naturally springs up within, obscuring what a loss actually feels like and what it actually means to the bereaved.

Rituals may even rouse the abhorrent stench of resentment and disgust, spurring the collapse of once-revered symbols as a society's individuals abandon its traditions, a violent reaction to, as Collins (2004) put it, "a kind of formality that one wishes never to go through again" (p. 51). So begins a ritual's slow descent into decay and irrelevance. And for the sake of many bereaved individuals who find compulsory involvement with vapid rituals to be stifling, these rituals very much *need to* be dissolved!

Personal grief rituals

Victor Turner (1967, 1969) understood rituals to be *an aggregate of symbols that gather meaning and transform over time*. They possess no static, inalienable function. Take, for instance, the evolution of grief rituals among the Zulu people of postapartheid South Africa. Upon returning from burial, mourners partake in a cleansing ritual in which they wash off dust from the grave site before entering the house, a symbolic gesture intended to leave grief behind. And yet custom dictates that the bereaved are to exhibit an outward appearance of misery in their grief and remain detached from the joys of present-day life for a particular span of time. Controversy and outrage have been stirring among the elders in South Africa as younger generations, fed up with the austere restrictions of tradition, have developed their own meaningful mourning ritual as an antidote to the gloomy conventions of old. Following the burial, family and friends of the deceased are invited to attend an *after-tears party*, during which all are encouraged to dance, drink alcohol, and consume food in a joyous celebration of the deceased's life (Kotze et al., 2012).

In his landmark pamphlet arguing for American independence from the British in 1776, Thomas Paine (2003) began *Common Sense* by writing, "A long habit of not thinking a thing *wrong*, gives it a superficial appearance of being *right*, and raises at first a formidable outcry in defence of custom. But the tumult soon subsides. Time makes more converts than reason" (p. 3). Cultural anthropologists who examine how rituals decay and lose integrity over time always turn back to the masses in hopes that society at large will engineer a new solution. The dissolution of one joint venture is to be replaced with yet another. But participation in the collective, however much it may be revamped over and over, is fated to place the same suffocating pressures on select persons within a society and choke the expression of their personal experiences of grief and mourning. The individual, it seems, must alter his or her behavior time and again to fit within what culture provides.

But what if this relationship between the individual and the ritual were inverted? What if the ritual itself, with its distinctive behaviors and meaningful symbols, could be altered to be in harmony with the individual? Rather than each member of a society waiting in bated breath for culture to change, the individual can endeavor to create a *personal grief ritual* endowed with personally meaningful symbols and sequences of behaviors that cater to his or her psychological needs and guide them through the mourning process.

The degree to which the individual benefits from performing a personal grief ritual *would determine its value for that individual.* Humans are too heterogeneous in personality, temperament, and life experience for a one-size-fits-all ritual to facilitate mourning for all members of a community. There will always be bereaved individuals who struggle to cope with grief simply because their distinct psychological needs require more or less of certain functions than what the structures of society provide: more or less expression of grief, a different emotional timbre altogether, an extended phase of liminality or a more succinct and faster clip that allows the bereaved to move forward, more or less adaptation to new roles, more or less ongoing and symbolic ties to the deceased. If willing to stray from the collective pressures of one's surrounds, the individual will be able to carve a unique path that guides them towards a more meaningful experience of mourning.

Nonetheless, an ongoing curiosity and open-mindedness about cultural grief rituals remain indispensable for the individual creating a personal grief ritual. He or she will be in pursuit of a more personal mourning experience that is deeply unique and private, but it is still misguided to outright disregard the wisdom culture has gathered from one epoch to the next. Perhaps the individual whose own culture and community, however familiar to him, has failed to draw out a healing process of mourning can look across the remote horizon and sustain his gaze long enough to discover that a part of his subjective experience of loss and mourning resides in the uncanny gestures, expressions, and movements of distant neighbors.

We have given much consideration to the vast topography of cultures across the globe and what they each have to say about loss and mourning. It is now time to direct our focus more towards the internal and psychological landscape of the bereaved individual. This will require a thorough understanding of how one person's thoughts, feelings of grief, and behavioral impulses after a loss differ from the next and how the unique bond the bereaved once had with the deceased determines the course of mourning upon which they are likely to embark. We must now move beyond the valuable insights of sociologists and cultural anthropologists, as they are not well-equipped to analyze the depths of a singular inner world, and turn to psychology to understand the many nuanced and subjective experiences of loss that reside within each individual.

References

Abruzzini, M. (2017, January 4). The Evolution of after-tears parties in South Africa. *Seven-Ponds.* https://blog.sevenponds.com/cultural-perspectives/the-evolution-of-after-tears-parties-in-south-africa

Becker, E. (1973). *The denial of death.* Free Press Paperbacks.

Birx, H. J. (2006). *Encyclopedia of anthropology.* SAGE Publications.

Bloch, M., & Parry, J. (1982). *Death and the regeneration of life.* Cambridge University Press.

Bonanno, G. A. (2004). Loss, trauma, and human resilience: Have we underestimated the human capacity to thrive after extremely aversive events? *American Psychologist, 59,* 20–28.

Budiman, M. (2013). *Contemporary funeral rituals of Sa'dan Toraja: From Aluk Todolo to "new" religions.* Karolinum Press.

Calhoun, C., & Gerteis, J. (2012). *Contemporary sociological theory.* Blackwell Publishers.

Carmichael, E., & Sayer, C. (1992). *The skeleton at the feast: The Day of the Dead in Mexico.* University of Texas Press.

Chen, G. (2000). *Death rituals in a Chinese village: An old tradition in contemporary social context* (Publication No. 9971525) [Doctoral dissertation, The Ohio State University]. ProQuest Dissertations Publishing.

Chwe, M. (2001). *Rational ritual: Culture, coordination, and common knowledge.* Princeton University Press.

Collins, R. (2004). *Interaction ritual chains.* Princeton University Press.

Doka, K. J. (2012). Therapeutic ritual. In R. Neimeyer (Ed.), *Techniques of grief therapy: Creative practices for counseling the bereaved* (pp. 341–343). Routledge.

Durkheim, E. (1965). *The elementary forms of the religious life* (Joseph Ward Swain, Trans. & Ed.). Free Press.

Farrell, J. J. (1980). *Inventing the American way of death, 1830–1920.* Temple University Press.

Farrelly, T., & Francis, K. (2009). Definitions of suicide and self-harm behavior in an Australian Aboriginal community. *Suicide and Life-Threatening Behavior, 39*(2), 182–189.

Freud, S. (1917). Mourning and melancholia. *Standard Edition, 14,* 243–258. Hogarth Press.

Geertz, C. (1960). *The religion of Java.* Free Press.

Giesen, B. (2006). Performing the sacred: A Durkheimian perspective on the performative turn in the social sciences. In J. Alexander, B. Giesen, & J. Mast (Eds.), *Social performance: Symbolic action, cultural pragmatics, and ritual* (pp. 325–367). Cambridge University Press.

Goss, R., & Klass, D. (2005). *Dead but not lost: Grief narratives in religious traditions.* AltaMira Press.

Grainger, R. (1998). Let death be death: Lessons from the Irish wake. *Mortality, 3*(2), 129–141.

Green, L. C., & Beckwith, M. W. (2009). Hawaiian customs and beliefs relating to sickness and death. *American Anthropologist, 28*(1), 176–208.

Hertz, R. (1960). A contribution to the study of the collective representations of death. In R. Needham & C. Needham (Eds.), *Death and the right hand* (pp. 27–86). Free Press.

Holloway, A. (2014, February 15). Turning of the bones and the Madagascar dance with the dead. *Ancient Origins.* www.ancient-origins.net/ancient-places-africa/turning-bones-and-madagascar-dance-dead-001346

Kerrigan, M. (2017). *The history of death.* Amber Books.

Klass, D., Silverman, P., & Nickman, S. (1996). *Continuing bonds: New understandings of grief.* Taylor & Francis.

Kottak, C. P. (2002). *Cultural anthropology.* McGraw Hill.

Kotze, E., Els, L., & Rajuili-Masilo, N. (2012). "Women . . . mourn and men carry on": African women storying mourning practices: A South African example. *Death Studies, 36*, 742–766.
Kubler-Ross, E. (1969). *On death and dying*. Macmillan Publishing Co.
Laird, J. (1984). Sorcerers, shamans, and social workers: The use of ritual in social work practice. *Social Work, 29*(2), 123–129.
Lange, C. G. (1912). The mechanism of the emotions. In B. Rand (Ed.), *The classical psychologists: Selections illustrating psychology from Anaxagoras to Wundt* (pp. 672–684). Houghton Mifflin Harcourt.
Laungani, P. (1997). Death in a Hindu family. In P. Laungani & W. Young (Eds.), *Death and bereavement across cultures* (pp. 52–72). Routledge.
Levine, E. (1997). Jewish views and customs on death. In P. Laungani & W. Young (Eds.), *Death and bereavement across cultures* (pp. 98–130). Routledge.
Lewis-Williams, J. D., & Pearce, D. G. (2005). *Inside the Neolithic mind: Consciousness, cosmos, and the realm of the gods*. Thames & Hudson.
Lexico. (n.d.). Ritual. *Lexico.com*. Retrieved August 29, 2021, from www.lexico.com/definition/ritual
Marcus, G., & Fischer, M. (1986). *Anthropology as cultural critique: An experimental moment in the human sciences*. University of Chicago Press.
Metcalf, P. A. (1976). Who are the Berawans? Ethnic classification and the distribution of secondary treatment of the dead in central north Borneo. *Oceania, 47*(2), 85–105.
Metcalf, P. A., & Huntington, R. (1991). *Celebrations of death: The anthropology of mortuary ritual*. Cambridge University Press.
Mitford, J. (1963). *The American way of death*. Simon & Schuster.
Needham, R. (1967). Percussion and transition. *Man, 2*(4), 606–614.
Neimeyer, R. A. (2002). *Lessons of loss: A guide to coping*. Center for the Study of Loss and Transition.
Paine, T. (2003). *Common sense, rights of man, and other essential writings of Thomas Paine*. Penguin Books.
Parkes, C. M. (1997). Conclusions II: Attachments and losses in cross-cultural perspective. In P. Laungani & W. Young (Eds.), *Death and bereavement across cultures* (pp. 233–242). Routledge.
Radcliffe-Brown, A. (1964). *The Andaman islanders*. Free Press.
Rando, T. A. (1985). Creating therapeutic rituals in the psychotherapy of the bereaved. *Psychotherapy, 22*, 236–240.
Rando, T. A. (1993). *Treatment of complicated mourning*. Research Press.
Romanoff, B. D., & Terenzio, M. (1998). Rituals and the grieving process. *Death Studies, 22*(8), 697–711.
Rosenblatt, P. C. (1997). Grief in small-scale societies. In P. Laungani & W. Young (Eds.), *Death and bereavement across cultures* (pp. 27–51). Routledge.
Santiago, L. P. R. (1993). The language of mourning and depression in Filipino and its Indonesian and Malayan cognates: Transcultural, sociological, historical, artistic, and therapeutic significance. *Philippine Quarterly of Culture and Society, 21*(3), 269–311.
Schnell, T. (2009). *Implicit religiosity: On the psychology of meaning in life*. Pabst.
Turner, V. (1967). *The forest of symbols*. Cornell University Press.
Turner, V. (1969). *The ritual process*. Aldine.
Van der Hart, O., & Ebbers, J. (1981). Rites of separation in strategic psychotherapy. *Psychotherapy: Theory, Research & Practice, 18*(2), 188–194.
van Gennep, A. (1960). *The rites of passage*. University of Chicago Press.

Walker-Gillet, S. (2011). Death: Indigenous and western views. *Undergraduate Journal of Native Studies: Dbaajmowin, 1*, 83–102.

Wilson, G. (1939). Nyakyusa conventions of burial. *Bantu Studies, 13*, 1–31.

Worden, J. W. (2008). *Grief counseling and grief therapy: A handbook for the mental health practitioner* (4th ed.). Springer Publishing Company.

Yasien-Esmael, H., & Rubin, S. S. (2005). The meaning structures of Muslim bereavements in Israel: Religious traditions, mourning practices, and human experience. *Death Studies, 29*(6), 495–518.

Chapter 2

Absence-and-presence

The subjective experience of loss, grief, and mourning

Mandy, an elderly woman whose husband died following a three-year battle with leukemia, talks aloud with her husband each night about her day. She tells him of how awkward retirement has been and that she has been able to nourish new friendships since he passed, though doing so has been a struggle. Mandy weeps as she tells her husband how much she misses him. Just as she had done the night before, and the night before that, she kisses the picture of her husband that still rests on his bedside table and says good night before drifting off to sleep alone in the bed they shared for forty years. *Does Mandy's behavior suggest that she has failed to accept the reality of her husband's death?*

Hank lost both of his parents early in adulthood. His mother died in a car accident, and his father passed after struggling with heart disease for many years. Approximately ten years later, Hank continues to feel that they are present with him whenever he achieves something of significance: completion of graduate school, a promotion at work, a marriage ceremony. There is no hesitation in Hank's voice when he declares that his parents are proud of him. And still, he gives voice to the pain of his grief and how he wishes he could ask them for advice about the next step in his journey through life. *Is Hank's continued sense of his parents' presence, alongside persistent feelings of grief about their absence, cause for concern?*

Emma is a young woman in her twenties whose sister died suddenly of a heroin overdose two years ago. The emotional toll continues to ring loudly as she remains angry about no longer being able to experience life with her sister. Emma copes with her upset by spending time doing activities they once enjoyed together throughout childhood. Whether listening to old music they both liked as kids or going on camping trips "*with* Addison," these nods to the past reawaken fond memories and comfort her even as she readily acknowledges that her sister is no longer at her side. *Are Emma's ties to the past indicative of an unhealthy and chronic course of mourning?*

Each individual's subjective experience of loss is an absurd and beautiful paradox. Fully aware that the deceased is gone, he still lapses into doubt when

DOI: 10.4324/9781351204873-2

attempting to comprehend a loved one's absence from this world. She cries and wails in defeat, having briefly conceded to the reality of irreversible loss, only to turn around and angrily demand that the dead return promptly. And even as the bereaved let go in due time, they cling with tenacity to an ongoing sense of presence, an echo from the past that continues to shepherd them forward. Such disjointed experiences of acceptance and persistent disbelief, sadness and angry protest, and absence alongside presence represent the pieces of a jigsaw puzzle that actually fit together quite well to form the gestalt of what healthy mourning looks like.

Nonetheless, questions abound as we strive to make sense of this complex picture. Why, after the loss of a loved one, do we not simply forge ahead with steadfast acknowledgment of the stark reality that people who once filled our days are no longer with us? We know that death will inevitably steal away our closest relationships one by one without discrimination; it should evoke no surprise and give no pause. And yet the loss of a loved one is met with shock. Death is experienced as an unjust and personal slight, as if the natural order of the world has somehow persecuted and betrayed us.

We are also left to wonder, Why is the emotional experience of grief so fraught with pain? Mourning is a self-restorative response to loss, a naturally unfurling sequence of reactions designed to accommodate death and adapt to life without the deceased. Still, it is a grueling process. Grief sends us reeling, grasping at straws as we fall into an unbearable reality. And it is not uncommon for this excruciating ordeal to burn for an unduly long stretch of time, sparking bizarre and perplexing currents of emotion that fan the flames of grief, often marked by persistent sorrow and yearning for a reunion we simply cannot have no matter how loudly we scream for restitution.

Cultural anthropologists assert that we mourn in the manner our culture dictates and that we do so in lockstep with fellow mourners to ensure social solidarity as the community faces hardship and transition together. This theory not only helps explain the numerous ways in which cultures express grief differently from one another but also fits with the psychological principle that humans turn to others to make sense of ambiguous circumstances and determine how to best proceed. The psychological notion of *social referencing* observes how a caregiver's affective response to stimuli is on display for the child's benefit, modeling the appropriate response so that the child can learn how to regulate their emotional response to stress. The roaring clamor of a motorcycle rushes by, but the caregiver's calm demeanor suggests that all is as it should be, and so the child, by proxy, remains unperturbed. An obnoxious acquaintance enters the house and leans in to talk to the child; the caregiver's lack of ease acts as contagion, and the child recoils alike in disgust. In mourning, so goes the anthropological perspective, reactions to loss are prescribed by culture, and individuals within the community, uncertain about how to heal thyself, happily take the medicine of suggestion. Members of the community exhibit their behaviors to signal to one another which emotions are appropriate, when their expression is encouraged and when restraint is preferred, and how long the state of mourning should last.

There is great truth in the observation that early experiences with culture offer explicit guidance about how to mourn, but it is a limited view. Such a perspective fails to appreciate the more profound explanation of why we mourn and why it is painful: We already know how to grieve from the moment we are born. John Bowlby, the father of attachment theory, conducted a vast array of ethological research to better understand the subjective experience of loss and grief. He contended that there is an evolutionary basis for mourning embedded within our innate, a priori instincts independent of what the environment prescribes. Humans, and many other intelligent mammals, for that matter, require no instruction in the matter of how to respond to the loss of a cherished relationship. As we turn to attachment theory to better understand how this can be, we find that the same instincts which compel us to hold on to loved ones in the first place also chart a course for how to let them go.

Attachment theory: Securing a safe base

Attachment theory is, quite plainly, the study of human relationships and the role they play in sustaining psychological health. It represents an extensive body of research on inborn patterns of behavior that help us form emotional bonds with our most important relationships and maintain proximity to these *attachment figures* (in the case of infants and young children, one's caregivers tend to be the primary attachment figures of interest). The degree to which these patterns of behaviors are successful in securing healthy and nurturing connections shapes the course of psychological development throughout the life span. Efforts to regulate emotions, our willingness to play and explore uncharted territory, the clarity of recall regarding past relationships, the manner and degree to which we lean upon others to cope, and the attitude that each individual has *about* their needs for affection and support are all set in motion during the most formative years of life. An adult may very well come to possess the capacity to cope and self-soothe when alone, but the germinal origins of emotional equanimity sprout early in childhood while still utterly dependent upon another's company.

Most adults continue to exhibit a strong drive to preserve relational ties, but an evolutionary perspective asserts that the stakes are strikingly high for helpless children, whose very survival depends on whether or not caregivers remain present and available. Remaining within the vicinity of attachment figures is of paramount concern. The child is preoccupied with as much: separation from one's caregiver is a grave threat to be monitored with vigilance early in life.

Young children relate to the attachment figure as a *secure base*, a reliable source of comfort whom the child trusts will be able to meet its emotional and relational needs (Ainsworth, 1963). The powerless newborn does not dare to venture away in the first months of life. But as children mature in due time, they master larger increments of separation – longer durations of time apart and wider stretches of space – insofar as they trust that the secure base will remain accessible upon return. She inches farther and farther out of reach before crawling back. The fledgling infant plays five feet away from their caregiver, then grows bold enough to play on the other side of the room. He withstands more minutes alone until he can no longer resist the urge to retreat back to base. These ventures away from and subsequent retreats back to the secure base of attachment paint a rosy and harmonious picture of human relatedness. But if we are to shed light on all that is mystifying about why the journey of mourning is so painful to traverse, we must take a deep look into the child's distressing experience of separation when time and space apart exceeds the threshold of what they can tolerate.

Panic in the nursery: Separation activates the attachment system

Children require space to cultivate their inchoate independence and master the fine art of self-governance. And they soon learn to find immense potential for joy in solitude and the unrestrained imagination of playtime when alone. But the ever-present need to be reassured that the caregiver is available remains paramount. Inevitably, separation throws a wrench in the works, and the child's slowly developing autonomy grinds to a halt. The attachment figure's prolonged absence evokes fear and inhibits further exploration. Such upset activates what is referred to as *the attachment system*, a host of behaviors designed to abandon independence, return to the secure base, and re-establish trust in its ongoing accessibility before resuming play once more.

John Bowlby noted that a child's behavioral responses to separation suggest that they intuitively know how to resolve the problem. Far from anything resembling a blank slate, children enter the world equipped with a battery of instinctual behaviors whose sole purpose is to increase their chances of securing and, when necessary, resuming proximity to caregivers (Bowlby, 1973). For starters, children know how to be cute from the moment they are born; they require no instruction on the matter. A quick flash of a smile here. An adorable coo there. Caregivers are helpless to resist the child's magnetism. The adult is drawn in to look at, interact with, and cradle such lovable creatures in their arms. Adorable little gestures serve as a preliminary strategy for reducing the threat of separation in the future, charming the caregiver just enough so that neither party wishes to part ways for too long.

Nonetheless, intolerable bouts of separation will occur, and when they do, infants are readied with an all-too-familiar attachment behavior: They create noxious noises. Tearful crying and frustrated screams induce distress within the attachment figure and beckon them forward to resolve the problem for both parties' sakes. In strict behavioral terms, the child establishes a pattern of *negative reinforcement*: Vexing sounds will be removed from the milieu only when the caregiver actively resumes proximity, thus reinforcing the latter as a predictable solution whenever the child wails again (the mechanism by which a car makes an obnoxious noise until the driver's seat belt is fastened works according to the same principle of negative reinforcement). It is incredibly frustrating to be within earshot of a child's displays of fury and upset, but its effectiveness cannot be denied. Infants in distress *will* get what they want. The adult may seek reprieve in sleep, but signals of distress will reliably smoke them out of their peaceful slumber time and again.

The child's emerging locomotive capacities introduce yet another crucial attachment behavior: the impulse to search. Learning to crawl and walk accomplishes more than lengthening the tether and allowing the child to explore the environment away from caregivers. Whereas the strategies already mentioned are essentially passive in that they entice the attachment figure to resume proximity, developments in locomotion provide children with the means to actively solve the problem of separation for themselves by pursuing the caregiver when too far afield. P. D. Eastman's delightful children's book *Are You My Mother?* tells the story of a newly hatched bird looking for its mother. The mother, absent at the moment of the fledgling's birth while foraging for food, is nonetheless imprinted on the newborn's mind, as is the instinct to find her. And so begins the little bird's myopic quest through the countryside to reclaim her nearness. These searching behaviors, characteristic of so many infants, may appear unduly clingy and preoccupied, but in fact, all is right. As Bowlby discovered, all these reactions to separation are constant across cultures and suggest something healthy is taking shape.

The attachment system is a brilliant apparatus, an intricate system of parts working together to strengthen a mutual desire for proximity between child and caregiver. The baby cries, and the adult grows fond of the tender exchange of affection that follows, not to mention the confidence that comes from being able to provide their little loved one with comfort. The infant is overjoyed to find mother on the other side of the house, forever endearing her to the child's wish to be near. The bond between child and attachment figure becomes increasingly reciprocal.

Many mothers and fathers new to parenthood are surprised to find that time spent away from their needy and demanding children leaves them pining for reunion. And for this reason, the child has one more strategy up the sleeve of her onesie: She wields small flashes of anger following prolonged separation. It is not uncommon for children to respond to the moment of reunion with a direct show of rage or a brief withholding of affection from the attachment figure before slowly warming up again. This seems counterintuitive. Why would a child exhibit angry withdrawal upon receiving exactly what it had wanted? This behavior can once again be explained through the lens of operant conditioning, but now the child is leveraging *negative punishment*, a punitive withdrawal of the very affection that the attachment figure has come to desire, all in an effort to send a lasting message: *Don't leave, or I will refuse you my love*. In the complex symphony of attachment between child and caregiver, the helpless infant is afforded a modicum of power in an otherwise-imbalanced struggle.

Failure by design: The attachment system in mourning

Audible transmissions of distress and the impulse to search for the attachment figure represent healthy reactions to separation. They are, as Bowlby (1980) aptly observed, acts of *protest*. And it was his singular genius to identify a meaningful parallel between the ways in which humans object to separation and the manner in which we react to the death of a loved one with reluctant demur. That a child's tearful pleas for reunion resemble those on display when someone is mourning is beyond coincidence. The bereaved are compelled to look for the deceased in old haunts just as a child is intuitively motivated to find the attachment figure from whom they have been separated. Within those behaviors designed to resume proximity to attachment figures lies the blueprint for how to mourn a loss.

Humans are irreducibly social creatures. As follows, the mind is hardwired to fight against absence, be it the impermanence of separation or the irreversibility of death. Both scenarios activate the attachment system. However, a cruel and ironic twist awaits when protesting against outright loss: The very behaviors that successfully resolve the problem of separation *are adaptively designed to fail* when the attachment figure is truly gone.

Ever the stubborn animal, humans do not acquiesce to death without a fight. The bereaved cross their arms in defiance, stay headstrong in pursuit of the reunion they crave, and scream louder in hopes that the dead will heed the call that beckons them to rejoin the living. But petulant cries and fits of anger no longer summon the caregiver to return. Efforts to look for and find the attachment figure turn up empty. Why would such a frustrating course of events prove to be adaptive?

Bowlby (1963) posited that unrestrained expression of protest is more than a stubborn request for an impossible reunion. Death and subsequent processes of mourning pull for the reactivation of attachment behaviors that, though ill-fated, are a necessary step in processing a loss. Bowlby insisted that:

> Open expression of protest and of demand for the object's return is a necessary condition for a healthy outcome. Such an outcome, it seems, requires the expression both of the yearning for the lost object, accompanied by sadness and crying, and also of the anger and reproach that are felt toward the object for its desertion.
>
> (p. 504)

Each manifestation of sorrow, angry yearning for reunion, and searching behaviors play an indispensable role in the process by which we ultimately accept and accommodate the harsh reality that *the other is no longer accessible*!

Loss is subjectively experienced as no more than another separation to be resolved, and so we engage in the exact same behaviors designed to resume proximity. The bereaved cry out in anguish and anger in a desperate plea for reunion, the unconscious wish being that the deceased will hear their cries and return to provide soothing just as they did in earlier years. We are equipped with the working assumption that losses are retrievable, that the people we love and depend upon most do not simply vanish; the lost relationship is to be rediscovered. From an evolutionary perspective, this underlying belief is highly beneficial for helpless children dependent upon being within the vicinity of stronger adults. But in mourning, the presumption that presence can be reclaimed proves terribly frustrating as the attachment figure is never to emerge from around the corner or be found in the other room.

Ongoing expressions of searching behavior are surprisingly common immediately after a loss. Many bereaved individuals report going to the site of a death or visiting a grave site in an earnest, albeit futile, effort to double-check and make sure their loved ones are not lingering there and waiting to be found, like some perverse game of hide-and-seek. They visit the deceased's old haunts, those places where the living were once reliably available. A patient of mine, who we will discuss further in later chapters, was struggling with the sudden loss of her father. She found it notably painful to go into her father's office, where he once spent the majority of his time. There was a genuine feeling of shock and surprise after realizing that she quietly expected to find him sitting where he had always been. The urge to deny time and search for him persisted for months, one unsuccessful hunt after another.

Brief nonpsychotic hallucinations may also occur: a fleeting mirage of the deceased walking down the street, or a quick echo of their familiar voice that sounds like it was actually uttered in the present moment. These phenomena express an intense desire to recover connection with the deceased and represent an abstract solution to the problem of absence. A contemporary example of searching behavior within mourning is found in the impulsive use of technology in hopes of communicating with the dead just as before. Many of my bereaved clients have caught themselves making phone calls to the deceased or attempting to make contact online through social media as if they could be reached by those previously successful means. While these and other behaviors of protest are commonplace and devoid of pathology in the early goings of grief and mourning, they are nonetheless *disorganized* in that they no longer serve their original function of resolving separation by bridging the chasm between self and other. Attachment behaviors persist with futility, and this is of utmost importance if the bereaved is to ever accommodate the reality of loss (Bowlby, 1963, 1980).

Literature and mythology are replete with stories of loss and failed efforts to push back against death. In the Greek myth of Orpheus and Eurydice, grief-stricken Orpheus is devastated by the sudden death of his bride-to-be, Eurydice. His intense yearning to be with her again incites him to traverse the underworld of the dead in pursuit of his love. Orpheus pleads with Hades, the god of the underworld, to allow Eurydice to return. The depths of his love sway Hades to bend his will and grant Orpheus's wish . . . but on one condition. As the two lovers leave the underworld together, with Eurydice following from behind, Orpheus is ordered to not look back at her lest Hades revoke his favor. Orpheus hears no footsteps behind him as he is leaving. No longer able to fight his aching urge to confirm her presence, he turns around to look and, in doing so, condemns Eurydice to remain in the world of the dead forever. His continued efforts to search ultimately render the loss irreversible.

The great epic of Gilgamesh, one of the earliest surviving works of literature dating back to 2100 BCE and born out of the Middle East, chronicles the adventures of King Gilgamesh, whose friend Enkidu falls ill and dies. The distressed king embarks on long and perilous travels in search of the secret to immortality, only to conclude that no such spell or magical elixir exists. His efforts to defeat death prove unavailing, and he resigns to accept his friend's fate, as well as his own. The epic of Gilgamesh, like the myth of Orpheus and Eurydice, is a parable about protest against the inevitability of death and the lengths we go to in our doomed efforts to deny death's inevitability and permanence.

Mourning proves to be quite the confounding task. Even our earliest achievements in cognitive development work against us when trying to comprehend the reality of loss. A child's acquisition of *object permanence* demonstrates this well. At some point during the first year of life – the specific time frame of this developmental milestone has been debated ad nauseum among psychologists – infants begin to understand that objects outside of their field of vision do not necessarily cease to exist (Piaget, 1954). Equipped with object permanence, the baby begins to search for what is no longer perceived at a given moment, and he will often succeed in finding a lost toy under a blanket or a marble that rolled beneath the couch. But this conceptual framework plays an unmerciful trick later in life when they feel compelled to search for the deceased; experience has taught them that all that goes missing is surely to be found if only they persist in looking harder.

The developmental achievements of *conservation and reversibility* also present unique conflicts. A young child eventually comes to understand that processes of change in an object, such as a solid ice cube melting and becoming a liquid, can be reversed so as to restore the object to its pre-existing state. This, too, sets us up for disappointment by suggesting that even if we accept that a death has occurred, the problem can somehow be reversed. Children will sometimes demonstrate that they understand a relative has passed, only to then ask when grandmother will be coming back again. Death is an insult to an entire system of behaviors and mental processes that allowed us to perceive the world more clearly and adapt during our most vulnerable years.

Furthermore, bereaved children and adults alike exude emotional distress because death is simply too difficult to fully realize. Psychoanalysts have long quipped that the unconscious mind cannot fathom outright nonexistence. Although we experience abstract approximations to death – loneliness, abandonment, or injury from an impersonal force of nature – we can never truly grasp the finality of death because it will remain forever beyond the reach of conscious experiences. This is perhaps why the bereaved regularly struggle to utter the word "died," preferring instead to mouth vague references to a loved one having "passed" or being "gone."

It is no wonder that shock and disbelief permeate the early throes of grief and mourning. Human beings are evolutionarily programmed to seek out attachment figures when absent. The cognitive development of object permanence imbues us with the working assumption that what we do not perceive within our perceptual range at a given moment still exists elsewhere, compelling us to search for what is no longer there. We also learn early in life to assume that changes in form, such as the living becoming deceased, might be reversed. From a metapsychological perspective, the unconscious mind cannot even take in the true finality of death! And what's more, philosophy teaches us that our subjective perceptions of the world, including our sense that those who die remain with us in some meaningful way, are irreducible despite the privilege that we try to grant to objective reality. The goal of mourning must consist of more than unwavering acceptance of death and of outright absence. Doing so, it seems, is beyond our nature. What, then, represents an attainable measure of healthy mourning?

Continuing bonds and the revision of attachment schemas

Protest continues in obstinate defiance of death, but in due course, the attachment system buckles under the steady and unforgiving pressure of external reality. The bereaved reluctantly ready themselves to accept that a loved one has died, but not before making one last stand. When a behavioral pattern no longer achieves its expected reward, humans will display a dramatic uptick in its frequency, referred to as an *extinction burst*, before the behavior ceases and succumbs to *behavioral extinction.* Misplace your keys and you look in the same place ten times before raising your hands in befuddlement and admitting that you do not know where they are. Discover that a file on your computer is not opening and you will click on the same icon incessantly before exploring different solutions.

In mourning, there is often a frenzied, last-ditch effort to reclaim proximity to attachment figures before conceding defeat. Emotional display ramps up. Forward movement is stalled. Searching behaviors carry on tenfold. As recalcitrant as one's protests may be, the attachment system finally gives way to the terrible truth, and the bereaved begin to gradually abandon hope that the departed can be found if only they looked harder or screamed louder. As Freud (1917) put it, "respect for reality gains the day" (p. 244). This is a good thing. The bereaved, no longer clinging to the hopes of a reunion they cannot have, may then liberate energy once invested in the deceased and redirect it towards life and those relationships that remain accessible.

And yet simply accepting that the deceased is no longer available is an unsatisfactory conclusion for many. No matter how much we privilege the cold truths of our rational faculties, we buck against the notion that mourning is merely a mechanistic termination of overt attachment behaviors. Yes, it is adaptive to stop searching for the deceased *in the external world*, but our gut-level reaction is to continue protesting. Frustrated with the constraints of objective reality and its incompatibility with our ever-present wish to maintain meaningful relationships with those we have lost, humans use their intellectual capacities and resolve this dissonance by rediscovering the deceased on a different plane of existence: the symbolic.

Humans have long made meaning out of an undying urge to reanimate loved ones in a symbolic form and rediscover them, as it were, in their surrounds. Bands of people throughout history have looked to the heavenly bodies in an effort to understand where the soul resides after death. They searched for their ancestors by craning their necks to find their spirits hovering above in the stars. The natural world seemed to burst at the seams with cycles of disappearance and rebirth that revealed their loved ones' whereabouts. People marveled at the sun as it repeatedly rose and fell, and the changing phases of the moon captivated their imaginations. The waxing moon was thought to be a receptacle of the recently departed as it filled with luminous souls, waning in turn as the souls migrated to an eternal life in the ever-present sun (Boorstin, 1983).

Bereavement may also fuel a drive to establish a symbolic and *internal* connection to the deceased. The concept of *continuing bonds* asserts that the bereaved maintain emotional attachments to the deceased; this notion has received increased validation from psychologists and thanatologists over the past three decades (Klass et al., 1996). This subjective experience of an ongoing relationship allows for a meaningful adjustment to the challenges of grief and mourning. The bereaved go on conversing with a beloved parent and derive comfort from such. They find great meaning moving forward in life with an illusory sense of the deceased's ongoing presence at family gatherings, while traveling, or during the culmination of significant achievements, such as weddings and graduation ceremonies.

Contrary to Freud's insistence that successful mourning demands the relinquishing of all energetic attachment to the deceased, there is no reason to believe that complete emotional detachment is necessary. Continuing bonds are devoid of inherent complications and can even be an integral part of healthy adaptations to loss (Worden, 2008). It is actually quite uncommon to find a bereaved individual who has completely dissolved themselves of a psychical relationship with the deceased. And the bereaved should seldom be advised to take such an inflexible course. Instead, the task at hand is to establish an enduring and meaningful connection to the deceased that does not hinder the pursuit of new life and relationships. As Shuchter and Zisook (1986) stated, there remains a place for the deceased in one's psychological life "that is important but leaves room for others" (pg. 117).

Humans do not experience grief and mourning through the numinal world of objectivity; rather, we perceive loss through the spectacles of our phenomenological experiences. A subjective sense of the deceased's presence is an indispensable aspect of how most people mourn and move forward. The three individuals alluded to at the beginning of the chapter – Mandy, Hank, and Emma – have all, in their own ways, managed to carve out room in their lives for healthy continuing bonds. Mandy's conversations with her husband at night lull her to sleep. Hank feels that his parents are proud of him each time he achieves a goal in adulthood. Emma enjoys the company of her sister while on camping trips. We do ourselves, our loved ones, and those under our care a great disservice if we neglect the importance of *presence* and insist that healthy mourning be hinged upon no more than objective *absence*. Nevertheless, we want to avoid the pendulum swing of implying that accepting the reality of absence has no role to play in healthy mourning. So how should the bereaved negotiate between absence and presence in healthy mourning?

Let us return to the Piagetian concept of conservation to demonstrate how the mind can embrace the paradox of something changing form and yet remaining the same. Early in life, the child is constrained by an inability to focus on more than one aspect of a situation at a time, what Piaget referred to as *centration*. An ice cube in the hand is just a cold and solid object. Place it in a container, wait thirty minutes, and the child perceives nothing more than water in a glass. The two moments lack a unifying link. But with maturation, the child achieves the capacity to forge symbolic mental representations of how their experiences change across time. Images of past encounters with an object are pictured in memory as a meaningful bridge between its previous state and the present moment. Piaget called this *the semiotic function*: An object or event that is present (i.e., the signifier) represents an object or an event not currently present (i.e., the signified). The child begins to associate disparate experiences of the same object across time. He comes to grasp that the ice cube, despite having dissolved into a puddle, still retains a watery essence. The mental representation of its solid state in the past helps sustain focus on that which has changed as well as that which has remained constant through the passing of time.

In healthy experiences of continuing bonds, symbolic mental representations of the deceased – the sound of their voice, their wisdom and counsel, the love and comfort of their company – serve to both recognize the change that death has wreaked while also allowing the bereaved to hold on to the essence of the relationship across time. The bereaved remain aware that the deceased is never to be found again in the external world; nonetheless, a symbolic sense of presence remains felt and meaningful within the mind. Has Mandy accepted the reality of her loss? Yes, and she continues to find meaning in talking with her husband. Hank derives comfort from a sense of his parents' ongoing warm regard even as he simultaneously remains saddened by their absence. Emma carries the felt presence of her sister wherever she goes, and these ties to the past aid her as she journeys forward in life, all too aware that she is exploring territory her sister never charted. Absence and presence can most certainly coexist in harmony with each other.

Beneath the system of attachment behaviors lies the attachment schema, a bedrock of basic relational beliefs and working assumptions about what to expect from interactions with important relational figures. The attachment schema maintains a mental representation of the attachment figure as a desirable source of comfort and guides the individual to resume closeness in the external environment. In mourning, an uninterrupted sequence of failed attempts at reunion ushers in crucial revisions to this schema that accommodate changes in the external environment, namely, the permanent loss of the attachment figure.

Mental representations of the attachment figure no longer represent a person to be sought out in the environment, whose absence activates distress and shuts down exploration. The bond with the deceased is transformed into something entirely different: *an exclusively internal and symbolic tie*. The revised attachment schema now guides the individual to seek out an internal mental representation of the deceased within the confines of one's mind. So much more than a mere storehouse of fond memories, the bereaved *continue to interact with their loved ones in meaningful, albeit illusory ways.*

Self-soothing in absentia: Transitional phenomena and object constancy

One of the most remarkable aspects of continuing bonds is that they continue to satiate attachment needs well after a death. Assuming the relationship was generally healthy and that the attachment figure was experienced as reliably caring and available, the bereaved carry on with their lives while still being able to seek out the internal representation of the deceased as needed. They might find comfort in maintaining regular, illusory conversation with those they have lost. When in need of reassurance during tough times, the living can access memories of a warm relationship that continues to provide support in the present moment.

Continuing bonds may result in the bereaved identifying with the deceased. Their valued attributes are internalized as a signpost pointing towards desired personal change, and the bereaved strive to merge with this idealizable representation of the attachment figure. Some psychologists refer to this subjective experience as an *ego ideal identification*. The bereaved strives to tell jokes in the same manner as their grandfather, contributes to charity just as the deceased had once done, finds meaning in a similar line of work, or derives joy from taking up a hobby, be it cooking or woodworking or a musical instrument, once synonymous with how the deceased spent their free time. Ego ideal identifications perpetuate a legacy while providing a feeling of kinship with those who have passed.

Continuing bonds may even come in the form of inanimate objects. Holding on to meaningful possessions once owned by the deceased offers yet another potential route towards symbolic connection to the deceased despite their absence. Touching an item of clothing they once wore administers a dose of tactile comfort. Cherished items associated with warm memories evoke fond remembrances. Jewelry infused with the deceased's ashes, an increasingly popular practice referred to as *cremation jewelry*, imbues the bereaved with a sense that their loved one is still near to them. Any discussion of the role that symbols play in coping with loss and mourning must pay homage to D. W. Winnicott's (1953) musings on the concept of *transitional phenomena* and how young children learn to manage separation.

Winnicott, a pediatrician who became a psychologist later in life, saw great significance in how young children become attached to blankets, teddy bears, or pacifiers as symbolic representations of their primary caregivers. His metapsychological theories posit that the mind of a newborn baby exists entirely within a fantasy of omnipotent control over its surroundings; oblivious to the mother's differentiated existence apart from the child's needs, the mere wish for the mother's availability is felt to create her presence. A cry, or a pang of hunger, or the desire to be held, he feels, is not believed to summon a separate individual, from another room, whose life does not revolve entirely around him. But no matter how attentive and quick the caregiver is to respond, the fantasy is destined to crash into reality as mother and father inevitably miss a beat. The infant slowly begins to realize that they do not have constant access to their caregivers. The objective reality of mother's separateness dawns on the child's mind as separation anxiety begins to loom (although this sounds like Winnicott was waxing philosophical, developmental psychologists lend support to his theory upon observing a spike in separation and stranger anxiety not immediately after birth but between the ages of six to twelve months).

Still yearning for control over the situation and frustrated by increasingly frequent lapses in the caregiver's presence, infants pivot to discover items in the external environment that can be cast as suitable stand-ins for the mother when she is unavailable. A teddy bear. A blanket. Even a thumb inserted into the mouth. Otherwise, run-of-the-mill objects are cast into the role of *transitional objects* imbued with an illusory quality as if they are meeting the child's original, most deep-set relational wishes. A hallmark of transitional phenomena is that objects charged with such symbolic representation do not enlist the child in an unchecked hallucinatory distortion of reality. The illusion is understood as such, but it *feels* real nonetheless; try telling a young child that the stuffed animal whom she has assigned a name and cuddled with every night for two years is *no more than* cloth, stuffing, and a few plastic buttons! Transitional objects are a compromised solution to the wish for actual contact with a caregiver, but reliance upon items within one's reach helps maintain a semblance of control over separation anxiety. The object of choice sustains the apperception, once belonging solely to subjective fantasy, that the comfort and reassurance that attachment figures provide are readily accessible when needed.

Winnicott noted that transitional phenomena are crucial to psychological development because they mark the beginning of a human being's capacity for self-soothing. The child exerts agency and actively ventures out into the world to get for themselves what was once passively relied upon entirely from others. And later in life, in the wake of permanent loss and subsequent grief, the ability to use transitional objects to self-soothe will be a deciding factor in the individual's ability to proceed through a healthy course of mourning.

Death is a blight on our spirits, too harsh to bear head-on. We need something to ease the bite of it. Symbolism plays an indispensable role in coping with loss and mourning because it provides an intermediary experience that lies between the harsh objective reality of loss and the subjective experience of nearness. The illusory quality of ongoing connection with the deceased, although understood to be a painfully insufficient replacement for the real thing, nonetheless manages to cushion the fall from presence into acceptance of absence.

In an effort to cope with loss, the bereaved seek out tangible transitional objects that represent the deceased's presence. The old item of worn clothing is so much more than mere fabric. The family recipe, passed down and recreated after its original cook has gone, provides something more profound than a simple meal. Photographs of the deceased and the stories we tell of our ancestors go beyond basic acts of memory. Intangible transitional phenomena deliver an abstract sense of connection through imaginary conversation, by means of aligning one's behaviors with the deceased's personality so as to identify with them, or through the experience of feeling as if the deceased is simply with us as we walk through life.

These efforts to manage grief through symbolism, whether we call them transitional objects or continuing bonds, are a product of the internal mental representations the individual carries within his or her mind. They bind us to a visceral past we can still touch while standing in the present, effectively straddling the fence between memory and perception. Most importantly, the comforts derived from internal mental representations and inanimate objects offer healthy ways to proceed through mourning while still acting on the impulse to search for, and hopefully find, important attachment figures residing within the mind. We may take it for granted that some individuals struggle mightily to do so.

Winnicott (1960) once famously quipped, "There is no such thing as an infant . . . whenever one finds an infant one finds maternal care, and without maternal care there would be no infant" (p. 587). Indeed, humans begin life enmeshed in a dyad that eat, sleep, and play together. Infants curl up in their parents' arms for comfort and rest. Toddlers clutch at the hem of mother's dress wherever she goes. Their entire being is engrossed in the task of staying close. But Winnicott's witty remark addresses something far more complex than mere physical proximity; it highlights how children are so psychologically tethered to their caregivers that they struggle to even *be* in the world and comprehend their surroundings independent of the relationship with their beloved attachment figures. The phenomenon of social referencing, referenced earlier, suggests that the caregiver acts as an *auxiliary ego*, interpreting the child's experience of the world on their behalf. The caregiver's calm *is* the young child's tranquility. How, then, does the child ever dare to go into the next room with their attachment figures out of sight, let alone march out into the world far away from home? The answer might seem to lie in a radical insistence upon independence, a wholesale severing of emotional bonds and ties, but there is little reason to trust that a complete jettison of dependence on others is a true marker of psychological health. Something else is afoot in the psychological development of healthy autonomy.

Margaret Mahler (Mahler et al., 1975) made it her life's work to study how young children manage the dual task of maintaining relationships with their caregivers while also affirming a separate sense of self; decades later, Sidney Blatt's (2006) research affirmed that *relatedness* and *self-definition* complement each other as interwoven measures of health. Mahler was primarily concerned with whether a child eventually develops the capacity to self-soothe when the caregiver is absent, and the developmental tract on which the child navigates this process is referred to as *separation-individuation*.

Despite the child's immense dependence on the attachment figure early in life, instincts pique his curiosity about the vast world beyond his narrow field of perception. As motor skills and coordination mature, a pull towards exploration drives him to step away from the caregiver and submerge himself into a world of wonderment. But Mahler observed that these earliest attempts, aptly dubbed the *practicing phase*, are destined to last no more than a brief moment or two before the child returns for comfort and reassurance of the attachment figure's availability. The child requires this *emotional refueling* before resuming exploration.

The most critical subphase of separation-individuation, *rapprochement*, begins between the ages of fifteen and twenty-four months. With each sojourn away from the secure base of attachment, the child musters up the courage to go farther out into the world and stay away longer. She is briefly oblivious to the caregiver's whereabouts, but the physical distance inevitably dawns on the child and evokes separation anxiety, signaling a frantic retreat from independence. The rapprochement crisis represents a conflict between the freedom of establishing one's autonomy and self-definition and the terror of losing access to relationships in the process. Should the child cling to an enmeshed attachment with her caregiver in hopes of securing presence, forfeiting self-definition in doing so, or – damn the torpedoes! – should she bravely assert her independence in larger gradations of space and time apart despite separation pangs?

Mahler's theory on separation-individuation tells us that the strains of managing separation go beyond a dichotomous choice between resuming proximity or leaving attachments behind. Rather, coping with absence demands a balanced reconciliation of the inherent tension between the drive to individuate and the need to remain connected. She coined the term *object constancy* to denote the child's emerging capacity to assuage separation anxiety by holding a symbolic representation of the attachment figure in mind (Mahler, 1971). Object constancy is a measure of psychological growth and the pinnacle achievement of the rapprochement crisis because it marks the beginning of an individual's ability to self-soothe at moments when others are not immediately available.

Most children resume explorations away from the secure base of attachment despite their anxious misgivings, but only insofar as they are able to internalize and access the nurturing and supportive qualities of attachment figures as a substitute for their actual presence. The child talks to himself and echoes the guidance of others in his mind, discerns between what to play with and what to avoid, and calms himself in the face of ministrations when no one else is immediately available to lean upon for comfort. The secure base of attachment comes to reside within and, according to Mahler, is interwoven into the very fabric of self.

Nonetheless, there is nothing quite like the real thing. The child can only lean upon the illusory comforts of object constancy for so long before yearning to return to the actual attachment figure. A young child is enthused to see her friends at school and play novel games, but when the bell rings at the end of the day, she happily retreats to her home to finish her day in familiar surroundings. She may leave her parents for the night to attend a sleepover and gush with excitement at the taste of freedom only to feel a twinge of anxiety in the morning as she eagerly waits for her father to pick her up and shepherd her back home. Assuming the secure base continues to receive the child with warmth, the temptation to go home remains throughout life. A young adult leaves home for college or tries his hand at independent living. He rejoices in liberation from mother and father's rule but periodically circles back to ease the ache of homesickness with yet another round of emotional refueling. He does laundry, basks in his parents' pride, and leaves again to explore more of the world. Many years later, the old man who has traveled the world and created a career and a family of his own revels in driving by his childhood home and absorbing the nostalgia of where his journey began.

A brief memoir of my children's rapprochements

Some of my earliest memories of parenthood are of me holding my newborn daughter in my arms and attempting to console her cries as I walked back and forth across our home. This was particularly difficult for me in the earliest months, when she was more attached to her mother, who would escape from the house for six hours a week to finish her graduate education. I marveled at how my daughter would actively search for her mother as we walked from one room to the next. She would cry out for "mommy" while turning her head this way and that in hopes of finding her. After a few weeks of these momentary disappointments, she learned to find temporary solace in our bond while still waiting in feverish anticipation for her preferred caregiver to return home. Four years later, on nights when my wife would sneak away to start her own business, our six-month-old son would wake from his naps to find someone other than his mother, me, hovering above his crib. Her absence activated biological instincts to resume proximity to her, and he panicked. He would wail in anger for hours, unable to calmly understand that his mother would be back soon. In due time, his protests lessened in duration and intensity, although they certainly did not go away altogether, and he, too, eventually learned to find a substitute comfort in his father's arms.

Once our children learned to mobilize themselves, they would seek us out whenever we dared to leave the room to grab a drink of water or go to the bathroom. They crawled into bed with us in the middle of the night upon waking up from bad dreams. And whenever one of us left the home for a brief spell, they learned when to await our return and through which door we would enter. When my daughter was two years old, she would position herself at the window near the front of our house so she could greet me at the end of a long day of work. And when my son was fifteen months old, he would point at the door through which his mother had exited earlier in the day and repeatedly say "door" until she returned, a rather-charming effort to exert omnipotent control over the situation and wish his mother's homecoming into existence.

As I finish writing this book, my daughter is now nine years old, and my son is five. I am moved to see their growing strength and trust in their own abilities to navigate the world. No longer anxiously tethered to their mother or me, they are content to run far out into their grandparents' backyard and frolic about with unbridled enthusiasm and thirst for adventure. My daughter is fully immersed in long days of school and sometimes spends large stretches of time on the weekends playing with friends or her brother or by herself in her room. My son participates regularly in hour-long gymnastics and soccer classes, where he plays not with his mother or father but with other children his age.

And still, I am equally moved to find that the ache for reunion remains among us all. On the evenings that my wife works, after I have put the children to bed, it is sometimes me who is the most eager to see her walk through the door. My daughter still reaches her hand out for mine on mornings when I walk her to school, and I am overjoyed when she opens her arms for one last hug before we part ways. My son, growing more comfortable with his independence every day, will stop halfway through his gymnastics classes to find me in the crowd of parents standing along the sidelines. He makes brief eye contact with me, waves his hand, and smiles before returning once more to tumbling exercises with his newfound friends. I suspect he has never known how much I, too, needed to touch base with him, if only for a moment, so that I could tolerate being separated from him again.

A safe harbor within: Object constancy in mourning

Object constancy helps manage the immediate stress of separation anxiety and, in doing so, ushers in vital lessons about how to mourn. Children first learn to internalize and access a psychological representation of the actual attachment figure during times of separation; an eventual reunion still awaits. But when the death of a loved one leaves us with no external relationship to which we can return, the internal mental representation of the deceased plays a critical role in regulating affect and forward movement. Outright loss presents the greatest rapprochement crisis of all as the bereaved individual is pulled in two temporal directions: an instinct to abandon novel pursuits and return to the familiar past, if only to grieve its absence, and a simultaneous pull to seize upon the freedom to explore the future.

In Mahler's framework, the maturing child learns to manage the rapprochement crisis and explore the environment away from mother with greater distance and gradations of time not only because they trust they can come back to the secure base as needed but also because the achievement of object constancy allows the child to retreat to her own internal mental representations in the meantime, a safe harbor within as the child waits for the storm of separation anxiety to pass. In times of grief and mourning, object constancy permits the bereaved to seek refuge in continuing bonds, an abstract, internal connection to the deceased that provides the comfort and internal strength needed to propel the bereaved forward.

Margaret Mahler's theory of separation-individuation and her notion of object constancy prove to be helpful constructs in explaining how most people are able to traverse the stress of mourning. The bereaved is most well-equipped if they can oscillate with flexibility between the spontaneity of exploration into new relationships and the ability to find solace in the familiar, secure base of internal mental representations. But not all people are able to manage separation and loss with such relative ease. It is imperative that we begin grappling with the reasons some individuals struggle mightily to mourn and cope with grief and why they are particularly susceptible to certain courses of complicated bereavement. Specific problematic outcomes do not occur by happenstance. They are a direct product of what attachment theorists call *attachment styles*, discrete categorical patterns of relatedness with others that form early in life. Our discussion begins with the exemplar model of psychological and relational health: secure attachment.

Secure attachment and the internal working model

Mandy, Hank, and Emma all serve as models for how to cope most effectively with loss. They each managed to process the pain of grief while simultaneously moving forward with their lives and maintaining meaningful continuing bonds. But healthy adaptations did not emerge as one-off responses to the stress of loss and bereavement. The trajectory of each of their journeys was set in motion long before their loved ones died. Their stories of mourning in adulthood lead us back to the opening chapters of childhood during which they had already learned how to explore their environments, how to grieve, and how to reunite. In fact, if we were able to travel back in time and observe their psychological development during the second year of life, we could reliably predict how they behaved in relationship to attachment figures. We would see Emma happily breaking away from her father, if only for a metered amount of time, to play and exude joy upon discovering new toys. Hank would surely express distress upon his mother leaving him alone in a room for a few minutes more than he could bear. And there would be Mandy as a toddler, crawling from one room to the next in pursuit of her caregivers and rejoicing upon reunion.

If John Bowlby is the father of attachment theory, Mary Ainsworth is surely its archetypal mother. Ainsworth and her colleague Barbara Wittig (1969) devised an ingenious research procedure that allowed them to observe a child's attachment behaviors in direct relation to a primary attachment figure and infer which attachment style best described the child's modus operandi for navigating relationships throughout life. The *strange situation classification*, as it came to be known, entails a scripted sequence of brief three-minute-long events which coax out different attachment behaviors under different circumstances.

To begin the procedure, a mother and child enter a room filled with toys as researchers peer into the room through a one-way mirror. This immediately provides a window into the child's *exploratory behaviors*, that is, his or her willingness to move around a novel environment and play with toys away from the attachment figure. Next, the mother leaves the room for three minutes while the child remains behind. This provides an opportunity to assess the child's *search behaviors*. Does the child follow the mother to the door? Does he orient his gaze at the empty chair in which she is no longer sitting? Researchers also pay close attention to the quality and intensity of the child's affective display in response to separation, be it tearful sadness, angry protest, or content smile. Lastly, the mother returns to the room. Their reunion is studied closely to determine whether or not the child seeks her out and derives comfort from resumed proximity. So as to assess levels of stranger anxiety, the strange situation paradigm also includes two episodes that involve a stranger entering the room when the mother is present and when the mother is absent.

A few key moments in the strange situation demonstrate secure attachment. First, the child is happy to break away from his mother to play and explore his new environment, but he does so without careening off into rugged individualism. He uses his attachment to the mother as a safe base to which he can return in brief increments for comfort before resuming play. Secondly, the child is noticeably distressed upon separation from his mother once she leaves the room. He cries, screams in anger, and engages in search behaviors, but all is well, as this emotional protest is indicative of a healthy attachment. And finally, the child is happy when his mother returns, seeks her out, and is soothed by their reunion; resumed contact is an effective solution to his woes.

Longitudinal studies that follow up with these children later in life show that one's attachment style in childhood holds up well into adulthood (Antonucci et al., 2004; Waters et al., 2000). Whatever patterns of overt attachment behaviors that emerge early in life tend to persist in relationships throughout the life span. The child with secure attachment will, as an adult, continue to express emotions in a healthy and reasonable manner. Her secure attachment will be evidenced by the ever-present desire for proximity to others alongside an equally strong willingness to explore her environment alone with ease. Like the child in the strange situation who finds joy in playing with new toys but also returns to mother with no hesitation, the adult trusts that she can venture away from others and eventually seek them out again should the twinge of loneliness seep in.

Attachment theorists speak of the *internal working model* (IWM) to refer to core beliefs about self as well as corresponding beliefs about the self in relationships with others. The theory begins with a simple observation: The vast majority of humans enter life with an IWM primed for harmonious interactions. This includes basic assumptions that (1) relationships are to be sought out for emotional support and comfort, (2) one's need for contact with others is essentially good, and (3) the pursuit of proximity to others is likely to succeed. Individuals whose earliest relational experiences predominantly confirm those positive assumptions are likely to develop and exhibit a secure attachment style fueled by an IWM that consists of both a positive appraisal of one's relational needs and a hopeful appraisal of the attachment figure's availability (Jacobsen & Hoffman, 1997).

In addition to overt searching behaviors, attachment style and its corresponding IWM are implicated in the degree to which adults can access early memories of attachment figures, effectively searching for relationships on a symbolic level within the recesses of the mind. Psychologists use an assessment measure called the Adult Attachment Interview (AAI) to ascertain the signature ways in which the individual *seeks out* these mental representations of others. The AAI reveals that those with a secure attachment express emotions about their earliest relationships with ease. They also recall memories in a coherent manner. Symbolic searching behavior abounds and is neither inhibited nor so all-consuming that memories of attachment figures distract from life as it plays out in the present moment. Furthermore, the retrieval of these memories miraculously continues to meet attachment needs. Remembrance affords comforting continuing bonds akin to the child in the strange situation who is soothed in the arms of his mother upon her return (Bifulco et al., 2002).

Just as early relational experiences crystallize into patterns of relatedness that continue throughout life, one's attachment style also has a tremendous impact on the subjective experience of grief and the course that mourning takes. Bereaved individuals with a secure attachment style are likely to mourn effectively because they hold themselves and their relational needs in positive regard. First of all, they can express grief and its emotional offshoots devoid of shame or restraint. Secondly, such individuals have typically managed to achieve object constancy by the time a significant loss occurs in their life, and so the illusory comforts of continuing bonds and fond memories can be leaned upon to ease the bite of mourning (Mikulincer et al., 2002). Third, they have learned to trust their autonomy enough to break away from the familiarities of old in order to adapt and explore the novelties of life without the deceased.

Let us briefly review John Bowlby's emphasis on the importance of sufficient protest. Those with a secure attachment style are predisposed to benefit from sustained expression of attachment behaviors that ultimately fail. In mourning, the attachment system is activated without inhibition because they have a generally positive and hopeful appraisal of their instinct to express distress and search for the deceased. These behaviors are *disorganized* in the sense that they are applied to an irreversible death as if it were a short-lived separation. The bereaved individual with a secure attachment system looks for his loved one in familiar haunts, cries out in agony, and shakes his fist at the sky in a futile effort to retrieve the dead. But their objections to permanent loss find no sympathetic ear in the cosmos, no permission to enter the land of the dead to reclaim their loved ones. These frustrations ultimately drive home the reality of absence and extinguish overt attachment behaviors in preparation for a future without the deceased.

But not all are destined for such a smooth course through mourning. Anywhere from 10 percent to 20 percent of bereaved individuals do not transition effectively through the challenges of grieving a loss (Bonanno & Kaltman, 2001). These difficulties coping with grief correlate with insecure attachment and antecedent struggles regulating emotions in relationships throughout life (e.g., Fraley & Bonanno, 2004; Wijngaards-de Meij et al., 2007). Ainsworth and her colleagues originally found that secure attachment encompassed only 70 percent of the child population (Ainsworth, Bell et al., 1971; Ainsworth, Blehar et al., 1978), and more contemporary studies of attachment style in adults estimate that approximately 58 percent are codified as such (Bakermans-Kranenburg, M. & van IJzendoorn, M., 2009). For the remaining 30 percent to 40 percent, the child's attachment system goes awry and paves the road towards a lifetime of insecure attachment, ineffective coping with loss, and complicated bereavement.

One's attachment style is either protective or a risk factor. Therefore, it is crucial that we understand the characteristic ways in which certain individuals struggle to cope with loss. We will soon contrast secure attachment with two different types of insecure attachment and how the course of mourning differs for each in notable ways. But in order to more fully understand the differences between healthy and unhealthy mourning, we must first consider one more theory: *the dual process model of coping with bereavement.*

Dual process model of coping with bereavement

Bowlby's attachment theory tells us that it is essential for the bereaved to express emotional distress amid mourning. They must tolerate the wrenching pain of permanent separation and make sure to not evade the process or repress any feelings. Bowlby's assertions might lead us to conclude that it is necessary to sustain the emotional stress of grief without interruption until resolutely expended and that anything short of this is tantamount to truncating the path towards healthy mourning. But a raft of research over the last two decades has cast doubt on this presumption and suggests that there is some value in avoidance.

Margaret Stroebe and Henk Schut developed the dual process model of coping with bereavement (DPM) as an application of stress-coping theory and an alternative to linear, stage-based models. The DPM offers indispensable implications for how to mourn and cope most effectively after a significant loss. Stroebe and Schut (Stroebe & Schut, 1999) identified two distinct types of stress associated with bereavement. *Loss-oriented stress* involves responses related directly to the death and subsequent absence of the deceased, often a loved one. These reactions include those typically activated immediately after a loss in order to manage separation distress: crying, experiencing sadness or anger, yearning for reunion with the deceased, dwelling on the circumstances of the death, reminiscing about the past, and relinquishing ties to the attachment figure. Loss-oriented stress is the stuff of grief work, those intrusions of thoughts and emotions about the deceased that require steady processing over time.

Restoration-oriented stress, on the other hand, pertains less to the loss of a relationship and more to situational changes following a death, what Stroebe and Schut call *secondary losses*. These stresses include those aspects of one's routines, lifestyle, and relationships left in disarray. Restoration-oriented stress demands adaptation to a life without the deceased that must be cultivated anew. The bereaved may have to tend to the loss of income, loss of physical intimacy, or altered involvement in a community. They may be embroiled in the legalities of settling an estate or of selling a home. The bereaved is often stunned by just how much of their identity and the roles they once played need to change in order to adapt. A widow must navigate the unfamiliar waters of attending social events alone for the first time in decades. A circle of friends will have to adjust to the stress of planning gatherings without the friend who had always taken the reins and filled their social calendars. A family member must open their home during Thanksgiving for the first time, filling in for the grandparent who had hosted for so many years. Whereas loss-oriented stress relates to what has been left behind, restoration-oriented stress entails what lies ahead (Stroebe & Schut, 2010).

The DPM flies in the face of any commonsense notion that the bereaved must move through mourning in a linear fashion, free from interruption, until they arrive definitively at a state of resolution. Loss-oriented and restoration-oriented stress present entirely different challenges to be attended to separately. But neither needs to be resolved entirely before tending to the other. In fact, Stroebe and Schut discovered that the bereaved fare better during the course of mourning if one stressor is dealt with while another is actively avoided and suppressed until later. This finding highlights *confrontation-avoidance oscillation* as one of the hallmarks of the DPM. The goal is to strike a healthy balance, with loss-oriented stress and restoration-oriented stress being managed in equal proportion. The bereaved copes with the stress of grief about the deceased while avoiding restoration-oriented stress and then copes with secondary losses as a distraction from the past. The bereaved spouse grieves for the absence of their partner at one moment and then must deal with the stress of cooking family dinners in the stead of their spouse, who had previously filled this role.

Failure to oscillate in this manner contributes to variations of complicated bereavement. Too much loss-oriented grief work yields emotional exhaustion, a lack of adaptation, and a *chronic* course of mourning. Excessive focus on restoration-oriented stress leaves grief repressed and unprocessed, leaving the bereaved susceptible to *delayed* bursts of grief or *masked* grief in the form of physical symptoms of stress and psychological bouts with depression, anxiety, or functional impairment in work and relationships.

Emma, Hank, and Mandy did not simply grieve without interruption until they moved on; they each exemplify a healthy course of mourning in part because they were able to alternate between grief work and adaptation to life after their losses. Mandy cried on a regular basis and maintained meaningful ties to her husband even as she was making new friends and navigating retirement without the love of her life. Hank was moving forward with his life after the numerous losses he sustained, but as he checked off one accomplishment after another, the felt presence of his parents buoyed him and evoked a bittersweet wish that they could truly see him become a successful young man. And Emma was able to express anger about her sister's death while, at other times, embarking on new journeys and adapting to changes in her career, her family, and her social life.

Bereaved individuals with a secure attachment style are able to oscillate between loss-oriented stress and restoration-oriented stress with greater flexibility and ease (Stroebe et al., 2005). The course of mourning is likely to unfold in a healthy manner if there is no inclination to lean too heavily upon one stress at the exclusion of the other. Regarding loss-oriented stress, the IWM of those with a secure attachment style appraises the need to activate the attachment system and grieve as essentially good and healthy. And restoration-oriented stress is approached in turn because the bereaved can explore the future while trusting that the memory of the deceased will remain accessible again when needed.

It is interesting to consider how this experience of healthy mourning mimics that of healthy play. The curious child feels free to explore her surroundings because she trusts that wherever she roams, home remains exactly where it has always been. Bereaved individuals with a secure attachment style are neither clinging to the past nor moving ahead unmindful of what came before. These individuals also tend to be able to meet the challenges of grief and mourning with object constancy fully intact; in lieu of an external figure to return to, they can seek out the compromised solution of an internal mental representation of the deceased. The illusory felt presence of continuing bonds comforts the bereaved as they continually orient themselves once again to the present moment and an external world the deceased no longer inhabits.

Complicated bereavement and the role of insufficient or excessive protest

Attachment theory lays out a story of how we hold on and how we let go. We enter the world imbued with an instinct to huddle together for warmth, and over time, we grow ever more attached to one another. The absence of our most cherished relationships stirs unease and activates the attachment system, a sequence of responses designed to resume proximity to attachment figures. Searching behaviors and emotional displays of yearning for reunion are grueling, but their inherent ache is indicative of something fundamentally right. If the pain of separation is sustained long enough to resolve the problem at hand, the individual encodes relational strategies of inestimable worth throughout life: Express distress to rally love and support, seek out others when lonely, and learn to tolerate inevitable stretches of time alone. Insofar as the child's attachment behaviors successfully secure reunion with the attachment figure, the child maintains calm faith in their ability to summon the other's presence in due time and resumes exploration of the environment alongside tolerable degrees of separation.

But not all will have such good fortune in their most formative years. For some individuals, frustrating relationships early in life derail their otherwise-healthy instincts. The child grows to doubt the potency of his efforts to pull others in. He may even lose faith in others, no longer trusting that the attachment figure will be reliably available. Neither able to fully fend for themselves nor depend upon others for support, these children learn that emotional pains are too much for them to bear. Attachment behaviors become warped into myriad disfigurements, tarnishing both the quality of their relationships and their ability to regulate upsetting emotions.

The entire attachment system is malleable: efforts to attract others, expression of distress when lonely, angry protest against separation, the impulse to search for others, the compromised solution of seeking out internal mental representations in order to self-soothe (object constancy), comfort in exploring the environment away from one's attachment figures. Each of these attachment behaviors can become artificially minimized or overemphasized, crystallizing within the individual's personality, and forever coloring the manner in which they relate to themselves and others.

For instance, some people do not make many efforts to attract others. They remain quiet when upset and refrain from bothering others with what they consider to be noxious emotions or bids for connection. They may even avoid the impulse to seek out others for support and insist on going it alone. Conversely, other individuals are perhaps too eager to attract the attention of others with a flirtatious smile. They do not discriminate when and with whom they cry or get angry, and they are compelled to seek out others compulsively, seemingly incapable of being alone. Either way, a distorted attachment system is a liability that only sustains the very emotional pain it was, in its unadulterated form, naturally designed to mitigate.

Bowlby posited that the behaviors necessary for mourning a loss are already embedded within the same instincts that help us build meaningful relationships from day one. Under ideal circumstances, the storm of grief and mourning activates the attachment system and draws out its entire range of behaviors. The impulse to express emotional distress and search is acted upon openly until the harsh reality sets in; the gentile tendrils of the attachment system reach out for warmth only to find that the deceased is not within its reach this time. And even as the bereaved let go and withdraw from hopes of reunion, they maintain continuing bonds and proximity to symbolic representations of the attachment, both external and internal. All this assumes that the bereaved will tread a healthy path.

But here, too, *the course of mourning is malleable* and can take various twists and turns. The entire range of healthy attachment behaviors – affective expression, searching behavior, and continuing bonds – may be chronically deactivated for some individuals. Bowlby (1963) advanced the hypothesis that much of pathological mourning is characterized by an inability to express the angry and tearful striving for reunion, rendering it repressed and unconscious. Insulated from overt expression and subsequent failure, the attachment system remains unmodified and persists quietly beneath the surface. But others still may suffer the opposite fate in mourning: the hyperactivation of attachment behaviors which never seem to expend themselves. Anger, tearful crying, and efforts to relocate the deceased are amplified and carried on without pause, unmitigated by time.

The attachment system is a compass designed to plot a course through the murky waters of mourning. But for those individuals saddled with an insecure attachment style, their compass leads them astray into calamitous storms. Each of the two types of insecure attachment style to be considered is associated with their own characteristic, patterned departures from an ideal path through mourning that lead to complicated bereavement. There is either an insufficient display of protest . . . or an excess of tears and anger. Searching behaviors are avoided altogether in a hurried attempt to move on and truncate reminiscences . . . or the search party is prolonged indefinitely. Emotional expression is either tamped out of awareness . . . or it bellows forth in a ceaseless surplus of pain. And according to the DPM, bereaved individuals with an insecure attachment style struggle with imbalanced confrontation-avoidance oscillations; their coping strategy of choice leads them to favor one type of stress while neglecting the other, like someone with an uneven gait who leans to one side while walking, taxing one leg while leaving the other to atrophy.

Additionally, both variations of insecure attachment style are associated with their own unique struggles regarding continuing bonds and a lack of object constancy after a loss. The illusory, symbolic presence of the deceased is either not sought out or it occupies excessive real estate within the bereaved individual's mind. One way or another, a lack of object constancy affords the individual no emotionally soothing connection to memories of the deceased. Absence and any lingering desire for connection cannot be navigated as if there were a prior context; the loss is subjectively felt to be wholesale.

As we step away from Emma's, Hank's, and Mandy's difficult but uplifting journeys through grief and mourning, we must now consider two bereaved individuals whose stories are more heart-wrenching and give greater cause for concern: Sabrina and Leroy. Both struggled mightily with the mourning process, but despite their similar circumstances, we will soon discuss how they each presented with markedly different complications. Sabrina's life ground to a halt following the death of her husband, and she spent her days absorbed in painful feelings of grief. Leroy also lost his spouse, but the years that followed his wife's passing were colored more by a cold, affectless devotion to work that was devoid of any real passion for life. Each of these individuals reveals a distinctive picture of what complicated bereavement looks like many years after the earliest years of psychological development have left their mark on patterns of relatedness and efforts to regulate emotion.

Insecure in mourning: Preoccupied attachment style

Imagine that you are a psychologist standing behind a two-way mirror and looking in on a mother and her child who have just entered the room. This dyad is one of many participating in your research on early attachment relationships, and you have seen remarkably similar interactions throughout the day. The mother and child remain close, but the child regularly mills about and plays with toys in the room. You then knock gently on the mirror, signaling the mother to leave the room, as was previously agreed upon, and the child grows upset. Searching behavior ensues: The child hovers near the chair in which mother was sitting and then checks the door through which she left. And upon her return three minutes later, the toddler calms as mother and child reunite in joyful bliss. You chalk it up as yet another example of a secure attachment; approximately six or seven out of ten will be categorized as such.

But the next mother and child who enter the room exhibit curious behaviors that deviate from the norm. You first notice that the child clings to his mother, and although this immediately strikes you as a simple display of attachment, it is soon apparent that the child hesitates to explore and play in the novel environment away from mother. He is certainly upset when his mother leaves the room, perhaps with a tad more intensity than what you are accustomed to seeing on the other side of the two-way mirror, but it is the child's reaction upon mother's return that grabs your attention. The child does not calm. Oddly enough, resumed proximity does not solve the problem of separation anxiety, and his angry protests persist with as much fervor as before.

In her research with the strange situation classification, Mary Ainsworth et al. (1971) discovered two distinct and patterned departures from secure attachment, each of which falls under the broad category of insecure attachment (an additional attachment style, disorganized attachment, was later discovered among researchers and found to be the result of chronic abuse and neglect in childhood). She categorized one such pattern of insecure interpersonal behaviors as *insecure-ambivalent*. Aptly named, one of its standout characteristics is that these individuals have mixed feelings about their most important relationships. They anxiously yearn for reunion when separated but remain inconsolable even when the attachment figure has returned! This attachment style in childhood aligns with findings from the AAI that codify certain adults as being *preoccupied*, and here, too, its title highlights one of its most defining features. Unlike the secure individual who feels safe venturing away from relationships because they trust that the other will remain accessible, preoccupied individuals anxiously monitor the attachment figure's whereabouts for fear of being abandoned (Wallin, 2007). They are consumed with separation anxiety. Preoccupied with ensuring the other's availability, they hold on to loved ones a little too tight and inhibit independent exploration.

Longitudinal research offers a glimpse into the fate that awaits each individual based on the attachment style they develop early in life. Children with an insecure-ambivalent attachment style are likely to upregulate attachment behaviors well into adulthood (Kobak et al., 1993). Emotional responses to separation are heightened. They will continue to err towards abandoning exploration and time away from others, narrowing their focus on finding and basking in the presence of friends, family members, and romantic partners. As much as they will be plagued by a crushing fear of abandonment, a deeper analysis reveals that they may remain equally terrified about whatever capacity they have for strength and autonomy. How could that come to be?

Research on interactions between children and their parents, the primary attachment figures in their lives, suggests that the parents of children who develop an ambivalent/preoccupied attachment style were *inconsistently* available (Green et al., 2007). Emotionally present and comforting at times, cold and absent at other times, the child learns that even-keeled activation of attachment behaviors does not draw out reliable access to the attachment figure. And so they up the ante. Where simple tears should have sufficed, a prolonged torrent of wailing and screaming *demands* attention. Rather than wade in the ebb and flow of closeness and distance, the child abandons play and hovers to ensure that the other remains nearby.

One of the greatest tragedies in this scenario is that the child comes to fear his or her own strengths, ambitions, and capacity for independence. They worry that any demonstration of such will invite the attachment figure to cease being available altogether, leaving the child to play and venture through the world alone. Autonomy and any genuine interest in being alone for even a brief moment threaten utter abandonment. Strengths are punished, and the child is incentivized to remain in perpetual crisis. The internal working model of those with a preoccupied attachment style is such that they see themselves as weak, feel dependent on others who are strong, and believe that they must amplify shows of helplessness through unrelenting searching behaviors and expression of emotional distress in order to ensure the availability of those who *can* shield them from the stresses of life and hardship (Kobak et al., 1993). But when the death of these depended-upon attachment figures rains upon them like so much hail, how do these individuals fare throughout the storm of grief and mourning?

Consider the case of Sabrina, a thirty-nine-year-old Jewish woman who came in for therapy two years after her husband, Sam, had died following a long bout of brain cancer. Sabrina began weeping immediately upon entering my office for the first appointment. I started, as I often do, by asking her to tell me about her relationship with her husband. They seemed to enjoy a fulfilling marriage and had two daughters, ages ten and seven at the time of Sam's death. Sabrina spoke of her educated, worldly, and successful husband with an air of reverence. She stated, "He was larger than life," and shook her head in disbelief that she had the good fortune to be paired with such a wonderful partner. She often deferred to Sam for advice about managing finances, world affairs, handiwork around the house, and so forth. But more than anything, she marveled at how much of a loving and supportive father he was to their children.

Sabrina was overwhelmed with grief. Bouts of crying ate up the majority of each day after her husband passed. But this seemingly healthy and appropriate expression of pain failed to ever expend itself or afford any fleeting sense of catharsis or relief; she only continued to drown in a constant state of sorrow. Uncertain about how to move forward without her husband there to guide her, she stood still in waiting and sought him out in various abstract forms. Sabrina visited Sam's grave site numerous times throughout any given week. She stared longingly at photos of him. And she was often distracted by memories of past conversations with Sam and the circumstances leading up to his death, ultimately finding it difficult to remain engaged in conversation with family and friends. Sabrina mustered whatever reserves she had to take care of her family's most basic needs. She and her children tried to stay connected to their community and did their best to take care of the household. Nonetheless, each day was an exhausting slog. The family home was preserved exactly as it was since Sam's passing: a memorial to their previous lives. The two children continued to share a room while Sam's office was left undisturbed. His books and the items associated with his many hobbies remained strewn about in their usual spaces. Sabrina reported feeling "helpless," and at the end of the intake appointment, she declared, "I just need a place to express everything I'm feeling."

Individuals such as Sabrina regularly find that the subjective experience of mourning is excruciating and unrelenting. Upregulated attachment behaviors yield a chronic course of grief marked by excessive yearning, ruminations about the dead, and other searching behaviors that persist unabated; the attachment system remains disorganized in a protracted state of protest. This is largely due to Sabrina's internal working model being saddled with self-doubt about her strengths and subsequent overreliance upon her omnipotent husband. She seemed to have been primed to respond to loss with panic and a heightened display of emotional distress in a desperate plea to reclaim proximity. Terrified by the thought of a future without her larger-than-life husband, she inhibited adaptation and exploration of life apart from him, conserving the majority of her emotional energy for efforts to remain close.

Complicated bereavement for individuals with a preoccupied attachment style often has the unmistakable quality of time being frozen, perpetuating an unconscious wish that nothing has changed and that the attachment figure will eventually return if only the bereaved stand still long enough and broadcast their suffering loudly enough. And so they wait in place, like a lost child separated from her parents at the airport. The bereaved posture themselves in a prolonged position of rigor mortis and refuse to move forward, all in resistance to the uncomfortable truth that the attachment figure is truly gone.

In Charles Dickens's *Great Expectations*, we find a poignant literary metaphor of chronic grief in the character of Miss Havisham. Although she did not experience an actual death, her life screeched to a grinding halt upon being stood up at the altar. Miss Havisham remained in her wedding dress every day in the decades that followed. She stopped all the clocks in her home at 8:40 in the morning, the precise moment she was abandoned on her wedding day. However unconsciously, Miss Havisham continued to wait for her groom to appear, and in Pip, she found an outlet for her rage, a whipping boy whom she could torture vicariously through her adopted daughter, Estella, as if Pip were the man who jilted her. Tragedy befalls those who stand still and stop the clocks.

Individuals with a preoccupied attachment style are further hampered by two antecedents to complicated bereavement: insufficient coping with restoration-oriented stress (Stroebe et al., 2005) and a proclivity towards excessive continuing bonds (Field, 2006). For those with a secure attachment, meaningful ties to a relationship with the deceased represent one of many components of healthy bereavement and can be loosened over time to also confront what lies ahead. But those with preoccupied attachment tend to maintain continuing bonds in perpetuity; there is little to no oscillation away from the past. They err towards confronting the reminiscences and yearning inherent in loss-oriented stress while neglecting the restoration-oriented stress of adapting to life after a loss.

Sabrina's struggles with grief demonstrate as much. Her thoughts and emotions are disproportionately directed towards reflecting upon the relationship with her husband that she lost. And in turn, she is hesitant to put those otherwise-healthy thoughts and feelings aside to give equal focus towards managing the stress of what follows. She basks in memoriam to the past but does not illuminate the path ahead. She lingers in illusory conversation with her husband at his grave site but only sparingly remains present when interacting with others in her community. Such excessive yearning for reunion and uninterrupted orientation towards maintaining abstract ties to the deceased perpetuate a chronic course of grief (Mancini & Bon, 2012).

Theoretically, a *lack of object constancy* is the most consistent culprit that muddles the pursuit of healthy continuing bonds. But how could it be that someone preoccupied by musings on the deceased find themselves struggling to access those very thoughts in a helpful manner while mourning? Object constancy is more than just the ability to resurrect memories from the annals of one's past; it is a boon to psychological development because it represents an ability to seek out *and derive comfort from* an internal mental representation of the attachment figure, a symbolic transitional object that feels real. The preoccupied individual can certainly conjure up memories of the deceased, but the subjective experience of retrieving these mental representations does nothing to mollify distress about separation and loss. Memories of the deceased amount to nothing more than echoes from the external world that the bereaved fear will dissipate over time. Just as she had been anxious about being abandoned by the attachment figure, in mourning as well, she is consumed with fear that time will rob her of memory, that the other's felt presence will cease to remain available. A lack of object constancy renders preoccupied individuals incapable of using symbolism to fill the void left by absence.

Here, too, abstract searching behaviors are hyperactivated in mourning. The preoccupied individual relentlessly seeks out the symbolic presence of the attachment figure in hopes of ensuring continual access within the inner recesses of the mind. She is myopically focused on efforts to monitor the other's availability, but such efforts provide no calming reassurance. The bereaved only remain in dread about the looming threat of further loss. Frightened to explore and direct attention towards anything or anyone else, the preoccupied individual sacrifices their future and clings to the internal mental representation of the deceased for fear that the symbolic will, in time, abandon them all the same!

The memory of Sabrina's husband remains fresh within her mind. However, she does not trust that his symbolic presence will remain intact should she venture out to cope with life after the loss. Hour after hour, she strives to continually rediscover him. Sabrina is stuck in a state of perpetual protest against Sam's absence. If ever her hyperactivated attachment system acquiesces to the painful reality of her loss, she will open her eyes to discover that holding tight to the past has left her unprepared to navigate the waters of her future, a boat tethered too long to a familiar dock.

The majority of our discussion about complicated grief thus far has emphasized problems stemming from heightened attachment behaviors: intense and prolonged expressions of grief, inhibited exploration of the future after a loss, and a preoccupation with memories of the deceased that fail to provide comfort. But we must now turn our gaze towards an entirely different brand of insecure attachment style that predisposes the individual to struggle with loss, albeit through a strikingly inverted course of complicated mourning in which the attachment system and its attachment behaviors are tamped down. If Sabrina's experience of grief was that of a blazing fire burning too hot and for too long, others find themselves mourning in a frigid and barren tundra, their skin numb to the touch as they check to see if they can still feel.

Insecure in mourning: Dismissing attachment style

By the time Leroy came in for grief counseling, his wife had been deceased for fourteen years. He was entering his late fifties. He spoke about her failing health and subsequent death with an unmistakably matter-of-fact tone, as if commenting on the weather. Leroy told me every detail of the rare autoimmune disease that had afflicted his wife and how she ultimately succumbed to medical complications that left her immobilized and confined to a wheelchair in her final days. Seemingly unaffected, he often shrugged his shoulders and said, "It is what it is," or, "What can you do?"

None of this negated the fact that Leroy clearly loved his wife. He regarded the romance and companionship they shared as the pinnacle of his life. Nevertheless, Leroy recounted how he decided to make a clean break immediately after she passed in pursuit of "a fresh, new start." He pivoted his focus away from the past and devoted all his energy to what lay ahead, particularly his business, which was a marked shift away from his usual relaxed and easygoing personality. Reminders of the past were deemed mere distractions to be removed promptly. Leroy jettisoned his wife's possessions. He committed himself to cease reminiscing about the life they shared for fear of being "stuck." He obscured memories of time spent together in their home beneath coats of neutral-colored paint, a far departure from the vibrant purples, greens, and blues that had previously adorned the walls, colors that his wife had preferred.

Despite his best intentions to move steadfast into the future, Leroy stumbled through the fourteen years that followed his wife's death, and his life lacked any real joy or zeal. Feelings of unease which he did not understand crept up while alone in his house, spurring him to work inordinately long days and sleep at his office. Any efforts to resume dating were quickly truncated. The women he met never measured up to the ideal of who his wife was; they were not quite as kind, intelligent, ambitious, attractive, or funny. Such comparisons compelled me to ask about his wife's personality, but Leroy, an otherwise-intelligent man with a sharp memory, struggled to recall many meaningful anecdotes about their relationship prior to her becoming ill. With a veneer of closure and acceptance, he repeatedly said, "Those times were great, but now they're gone."

Mary Ainsworth's research identified an entirely different category of insecure attachment style in children called *insecure-avoidant* that aligns with patterns of relational behavior in adulthood that the AAI codes as *dismissing*. Its key characteristic is that the individual presents with a cool demeanor of indifference in relation to other people. Relationships, whether present or not, seem to be of little concern. They adopt a "take it or leave it" attitude, content to interact with others at times, but devoid of feelings of loneliness or any pining for reunion when alone.

Now, use your imagination once again to place yourself behind the two-way mirror and envision what it would be like to watch Leroy navigate the strange situation as a toddler. Like so many avoidant children, you would first notice that he is all too eager to explore the room and play with toys. This initial behavior might suggest secure attachment, but something curious and concerning unfolds as the minutes pass. The child remains perfectly content playing by himself and rarely returns to his mother for comfort. Exploration is abnormally high. And when the mother leaves the room, the child is indifferent to her absence. He continues to play on his own. Separation seems to register as a non-event, and when the mother returns, there is no noticeable drive to connect. Independent exploration continues without interruption.

Avoidant/dismissing attachment is tricky to detect because the individual's unperturbed calm suggests that all is well, that the child is exhibiting inner strength and a mature capacity for independence. This is especially the case within individualistic cultures that pride themselves on self-sufficiency. Even students of psychology regularly jump to the conclusion that this kind of presentation indicates healthy and secure attachment. Although this constellation of behaviors may masquerade as contentment and autonomy, something insidious is festering within. Research on children with avoidant attachment reveals that as much as they present a veneer of serenity, nonetheless, physiological symptoms of distress persist beneath the surface when separated from attachment figures (Hill-Soderlund et al., 2008; Sroufe & Waters, 1977). Heart rate soars. Levels of cortisol, a hormone implicated in stress responses, shoot through the roof. Some medical research (Kotler et al., 1994) suggests that children with avoidant attachment are more susceptible to stress-induced illness because they have effectively abandoned emotional expression and the pursuit of interpersonal support as hard-wired solutions to separation distress. If preoccupied attachment is a loud and explosive demand for the other to return, dismissing attachment is a slow and quiet meltdown.

A child who exhibits an avoidant attachment style will likely perpetuate a pattern of downregulated attachment behaviors well into adulthood. He will often prefer to go it alone and explore the world untethered to other people. Searching behavior has been largely deactivated, and so relationships are not regularly sought out when distressed. Expression of emotional distress also tends to be kept at bay, as responses to separation from those they have allowed into their lives are minimized: Separation anxiety does not register on the Richter scale. Here, too, we are left to wonder how this could have come to be.

Research suggests that early child-parent interactions suffered from either too much availability or too little. When the child activated attachment behaviors, they either elicited an overwhelming level of responsiveness that smothered the child's autonomy or a dearth of such that left them abandoned. Whichever extreme is encountered, the result is the same: These children begin to cast aside their attachment behaviors as undesirable liabilities.

The excessively available mother responds to *every* cry. She is *always* there, suffocating the child's drive to occasionally explore the environment alone. The child learns that shutting down affect will afford some room to play without the hovering presence of supervision cramping their space. Conversely, the insufficiently available parent who rarely, if ever, responds to distress imbues the child with *learned helplessness*. That is, the child concludes that it is pointless to exert energy pursuing relational needs because doing so fails to yield a helpful result and only disappoints.

When attachment is secure, the individual gives equal weight to independent exploration and the drive to ensure proximity to others. These disparate needs coexist in a harmonious ebb and flow where one takes precedence for a time until gracefully receding to give way to the other. But the child with an insecure-avoidant attachment style begins to disproportionately favor independence over connection. He regularly withdraws from others. And in adulthood, the dismissing individual finds himself firmly entrenched in a pattern of giving himself all that he had originally hoped others could provide.

The internal working model of those with a dismissing attachment style appraises one's own efficacy as positive, though self-esteem is not necessarily high, as a history of being rejected by caregivers leaves them feeling undeserving of love (Larose & Bernier, 2001). Others are generally expected to be unavailable, but to the extent that they *are* available, it is assumed they will impinge or be outright unhelpful. Either way, efforts to enlist the support of other adults to cope are perceived as futile. Searching behaviors and the impulse to express distress are buried and remain repressed, even during times of loss and grief.

Although the circumstances of Sabrina's and Leroy's losses were largely the same, his particular struggles present an entirely different picture of what complicated bereavement can look like. For those with a dismissing attachment style, the immediate subjective experience of loss often appears unremarkable. They seem to adapt to the reality of loss and resume busying themselves with life after a death without lingering over difficult feelings. But the pain of grief is unforgiving in its relentless push for expression. Like a crack in a dam submitting to forces beyond its strength, the weary psyche is bound to buckle under the pressure of grief it has failed to vent. Thoughts, feelings, and behavioral impulses can only be held back for so long and, if not given expression in due time, are destined to eventually burst forth in a destructive cascade.

Downregulated attachment behaviors place the bereaved individual in a precarious position, as the debt of unprocessed grief is eventually paid during a *delayed* or *masked* course of mourning. Searching behavior and expression of distress do not abate simply because they are ignored. Never having been properly acted upon, the true depths of their pain fester and find a path of least resistance through obscure psychological ailments and problematic patterns of behavior that may not show up until well after a death has occurred.

Leroy tried in earnest to bury his grief beneath restoration-oriented distractions. He attempted to shut out reminiscences about the past or any other efforts to remain connected to the memory of his wife. But protest reared its head through uncomfortable feelings while in his home and inhibitions while dating. These problems persisted for years largely because he did not regard them as having any meaningful tie to grief. It is quite common for bereaved individuals like Leroy to seek out professional help many years after a significant loss, perplexed about why they have sabotaged their career, why their health has succumbed to symptoms of stress, or why they have been stuck in a pattern of unfulfilling relationships.

Those with a dismissing attachment style are prone to complicated bereavement because of two additional factors: insufficient coping with loss-oriented stress (Stroebe et al., 2005) and a dearth of continuing bonds (Field, 2006). Whereas some bereaved individuals are too tethered to the past, others are too quick to cut the cord and move forward. In terms of the DPM, they lean too much into restoration-oriented stress. They focus their gaze on the stresses of adapting to life after a death future without pausing to look back and emote about what has been lost. And if the bereaved fail to cope with grief for too long, a neglected past still looms in the psyche, threatening to rear its head and wreak havoc at inopportune times.

Furthermore, a general aversion to continuing bonds also leaves the bereaved unable to derive comfort through memory or an illusory sense of felt presence. This is largely due to a lack of object constancy, albeit markedly different from what is observed in individuals with a more preoccupied attachment style. Some scholars have noted that avoidant/dismissing attachment involves minimization of negative emotions and *an absence of cognitive access to thoughts of attachment figures* (Meier et al., 2013). The adult who does not regularly seek out memories of important relationships will deactivate abstract searching behaviors in mourning that could have helped them cope. One of the more interesting findings from studies with the AAI is that individuals with a dismissing attachment style, whose minds are otherwise sound, struggle to recall meaningful memories of their attachment figures (Meier et al., 2013). Far from a case of organic amnesia, the symbolic mental representation of the deceased does live on internally but is tucked away in such remote corners of the mind that the bereaved have trouble coaxing it out.

Loss-oriented stress and continuing bonds alike are consistently avoided amid the mourning process if early experiences primed the bereaved to doubt whether any good will come from expressing separation distress or pursuing abstract connections. Activation of the attachment system, they fear, would be a shame-filled admission of dependence that threatens their hard-fought sense of independence. Thus, any impulse to find comfort in continuing bonds or search for the deceased by sifting through memory is swiftly swept under the rug.

Bereaved individuals like Leroy posture as if they are content being alone, and yet they are dying a slow death of desperate loneliness. The urge to reunite lives on within the deepest strata of the mind. It lies in wait for an opportunity to be voiced. But if muzzled for too long, it manifests in thwarted efforts to move forward and the pursuit of problematic relationships that only obscure their true yearning for reunion with the deceased. There seems to be a hitch in each step they try to take. The bereaved may postpone the sale of their parents' house for years as a discreet wish to return home and find mother waiting there. Expression of distress, if not channeled through verbal statements of grief and conscious acts of mourning, will gain expression through indirect displays of upset: anxiety, poor sleep, irritability, and efforts to circumvent needs for interpersonal comfort with self-administered drug abuse or consumption of unhealthy food.

As much as Leroy tried to bury his grief under coats of paint, uncomfortable feelings bubbled up while in the home and sent him fleeing to distract himself in work. And despite efforts to keep his wife out of mind, he could never enjoy the companionship of a woman who was actually in his presence, because he seemed to be looking for a reincarnation of his wife's personality in someone else. The dismissing individual risks living out their days haunted by ghosts whom they never said goodbye to.

Negative continuing bonds: The slippery slope of symbolism

As much as continuing bonds carry immense potential to ease the pain of adapting to life after a loss, they prove to be a hard-fought reward for having properly mourned. One must tolerate the emotional turmoil of grief until sufficient confrontation with absence gives way to the compromised solution of symbolic presence. One's subjective experience of the other's nearness must manage to exist alongside the stark truth that the other is not there. Only then can the bereaved strike a balance between playing out illusory interactions with the deceased and then venturing away for a while to attend to present day relationships. They can seek out the symbolic mental representation of the deceased *and* separate from it. But symbolization of the dead can be a slippery slope.

Sabrina's uninterrupted thoughts of her husband represent an abstract interaction that shields her from acknowledging the pain that he is truly gone. Leroy has simply avoided reflecting upon his wife and, in doing so, has robbed himself of the opportunity to find an enduring place for her within his heart and mind as he moves forward. Though their struggles are starkly different from one another, Sabrina and Leroy each demonstrate a course of complicated bereavement marked by *negative continuing bonds*.

Negative continuing bonds are essentially a problem of inadequate separation. Some bereaved individuals, like Sabrina, exhaust themselves in continual pursuit of reassurance that memories of the deceased remain just as available as before. For others, like Leroy, stepping away from the inner recesses of the mind and out into their surrounds is done only in service of unconsciously searching for the deceased in effigy. This is evident in myriad examples of outmoded attachment behaviors which obscure the reality of absence.

Mummification, for instance, refers to the meticulous maintenance of living spaces exactly as they were prior to a death (Gorer, 1965). This expression of negative continuing bonds is fueled by a fantasy that no time has passed, that nothing has changed, and that the relationship will pick up where it left off upon the deceased's return. Bedrooms, offices, and other places the deceased once frequented are watched over and preserved, kept perfectly intact to receive them upon homecoming. Sabrina, in many ways, maintained the house just as it was so that her husband would recognize it should he spontaneously materialize.

Substitutes entail a hungry search for others who can fill the relational void left vacant after a death. They amount to distorted perceptions, what Bowlby (1980) called mislocation: New relationships are used as stand-in replacements of the deceased. In doing so, the bereaved not only do themselves a disservice but also struggle to respect the other's separate identity, essentially an act of objectification. It is quite common for the bereaved to grow frustrated should the other behave differently than the dead. Leroy, for instance, was often dissatisfied when dating women because they inevitably failed to be a carbon copy replica of his wife.

One form of negative continuing bonds that deserves special consideration is referred to as *linking objects*. Though similar to transitional objects, differences between the two highlight important distinctions between healthy and complicated bereavement. Transitional objects are associated with positive continuing bonds. In infancy, the parent leaves the room for an uncomfortable stretch of time and the child manages subsequent separation anxiety by finding, if you will, his mother in the warm, tactile comfort of a teddy bear. Later in life, the bereaved adult can lean upon transitional objects that provide a comforting sense of ongoing connection to the deceased while also ushering in incremental awareness of loss so that mourning can unfurl at a manageable pace that does not overwhelm. Grief is not fended off entirely.

Winnicott insisted that the blanket or teddy bear is not supposed to outright supplant the attachment figure. The object, too, is destined to be relinquished in due time. While there is room to argue that continuing bonds to the deceased need not be renounced entirely, nonetheless, the energy once invested in those abstract ties does tend to lessen to some degree as mourning progresses.

These otherwise-healthy continuing bonds can devolve into insidious linking objects if fantasy is not sufficiently tempered by reality. Linking objects play on a similar impulse to maintain symbolic ties to important figures, but the illusory connection only serves to avoid feelings of grief, exert omnipotent control, and deny the reality of loss altogether, giving way to what Vamik Volkan (1972) called *established pathological mourning*. A variety of tangible items associated with the deceased can become problematic linking objects: personal possessions, clothing once worn by the deceased, objects connected to their hobbies, photographs, something symbolic of the relationship, or an item associated with the event of the death. But linking objects are no mere keepsakes. Inanimate items become animated with the deceased's ongoing presence in a defiant act of delusional protest and preservation. The experience of becoming attached to linking objects lacks conscious acknowledgment that the item merely represents what has been lost.

Outside parties may be hesitant to discourage this behavior for fear of ripping away the individual's only vestige of ongoing connection, but it is worth noting that linking objects rarely provide actual comfort and soothing. The telltale sign that such an item contributes to pathological mourning is that its whereabouts are anxiously monitored. Volkan observed that the linking object comes to represent the actual body of the deceased, and grief ensues only if the item is misplaced. Thus, the motivation for clinging to linking objects is laid bare: to fend off the reality of the loss, feelings of grief, and modification of the attachment schema. This theoretical construct helps to explain why it is so common for bereaved individuals to struggle with hoarding behaviors after a loss. The subjective experience of surrounding oneself with relics of a past relationship regularly reveals an elaborate instinct to preserve items that represent the deceased and, in doing so, protect the valued relationship and shield oneself from the full brunt of grief. I have helped many bereaved clients let go of superfluous items they have held on to within their home after a loss and witnessed, with awe, the intense emotions usually reserved for acute reactions to loss burst forth, sometimes years after the actual death occurred.

While some inanimate items can surely play a role in healthy mourning, linking objects denote a failure to consciously symbolize the lost relationship. The item does not simply remind them of the past relationship or evoke a meaningful connection that meets attachment needs; the item is related to *as if it were the deceased*. Naturally, like a shipwrecked sailor clutching a leaky raft, the deceased is quite reluctant to part with their linking objects. Linking objects are negative continuing bonds in that they involve disorganized attachment behaviors, distorted efforts to maintain proximity to loved ones through things.

The phenomena of mummification, substitutes, and linking objects all belong to a category of unhealthy searching behaviors that occur in the external environment. But negative continuing bonds can also play out in the internal spaces of the psyche. Dating back to Sigmund Freud (1917), psychoanalytic psychologists have referred to *introjects* as the subjective experience of another person's presence within the mind, and these introjects contribute mightily to complicated bereavement when they are intrusive and unwanted. This immediately sounds like the stuff of a psychotic episode, but those who are of otherwise-sound mind may sense that a deceased parent or spouse continues to lord over them. The dead seem to cast judgment from beyond the grave. And the bereaved may even find themselves identifying with and behaving in unsavory ways like the person they lost, disturbed by the feeling that the other's personality has infiltrated their own. Lastly, those embroiled in chronic grief and mourning may feel driven to continue meeting the deceased individual's needs and expectations as if they were still present, thinking or behaving in a manner that once elicited approval or fended off criticism.

Despite Leroy's limited efforts to retrieve conscious memories of his wife, it eventually became apparent that she valued hard work above all else and that she often overexerted herself at her job to the point where she would . . . sleep at her office. She would gently poke fun at Leroy's laid-back persona with thinly veiled disapproval; conversely, she championed him whenever he pushed himself to work harder at his business than usual. Is it beyond coincidence that Leroy's personality took a shift after his wife's death and that he aligned his work ethic with her industriousness? Might Leroy's attempts to cope with grief by drowning himself in work represent an unconscious yearning to keep her memory alive by incorporating her essence into his own?

Negative continuing bonds are maladaptive in that the bereaved is driven to remain close but fails to appreciate that the deceased exists only at the internal, representational level. There would be no cause for concern if Leroy exhibited a conscious desire to honor his wife's memory by embodying her attitude towards hard work. This would, in fact, be a healthy continuing bond. But instead, he was propelled forward by implicit motives he was neither acknowledging nor processing, leaving him blocked off to companionship and fleeing his home to bury grief in excessive work. It would be quite healthy for Sabrina to confront the pain of slowly rearranging Sam's office while also maintaining some corners in the house where she and her children could hold on to mementos that remind them of his presence. But here, too, Sabrina preserved the house just as it was and ultimately struggled to adapt to the present moment. All these cases serve as cautionary tales of what happens when the bereaved fail to balance the desire to hold on with the necessity of letting go.

Absence-and-presence

The subjective experience of loss is a complex tapestry of acceptance and persistent protest, retreat to the past and exploration of the future, dreadful loneliness and the near-magical comforts of continuing bonds. Mourning entails a process of navigating this storm of pain and healing. The bereaved instinctively misconstrues death as a mere separation to be resolved. Separation anxiety mobilizes attachment behaviors that act on a presumed ability to retrieve the other, but these once-helpful instincts are fated to fail. Crying, angry yearning for reunion, and searching behaviors all give way to the dreaded realization that the attachment figure remains forever absent.

It is popular to quip that mourning never truly ends, but I find it unhelpful to dispense such equivocation. This noncommittal sentiment likely stems from the trap of conflating the pain of grief with the process of mourning. As much as grief may continue to erupt throughout life, mourning is nonetheless a self-restorative process that should effectively accommodate reality and help the bereaved adapt to life without the deceased. But still, there is more to mourning than straightforward acceptance of death.

Amid the strains of grief for what has been lost (loss-oriented stress) and the exacting efforts to cope with all that has changed (restoration-oriented stress), symbolic searching behaviors persist in defiance of external reality. The instinct to seek out absent attachment figures is reconstituted as an internal endeavor within the mind where the deceased may, in a sense, be found. Positive continuing bonds emerge under healthy conditions that afford the bereaved a compromised semblance of the deceased's presence. Yes, we are to accept loss for what it plainly is: the *absence* of someone who was once here. We aspire to express emotions in line with the pain of such. And the attachment schema that once guided the individual to seek out a particular person must be revised to no longer expect that contact will be available in the external world. But we must not overlook the fact that rediscovering the other's *presence* and availability at an internal level also has its place in healthy mourning. This immediately stings of paradox: Are we to both hold on and let go? I argue that this is precisely the stuff of healthy mourning.

Let us recall the three cases discussed at the beginning of the chapter. An understanding of mourning that disproportionately privileges objective absence would lead us to conclude that Mandy, Hank, and Emma are all failing to cope with reality, that their experiences of interacting with the deceased are indicative of denial and delusion. Yet each of these individuals has accommodated the reality of their losses and is living a meaningful and happy life in part because of their continuing bonds. Mandy, the older woman who speaks with her deceased husband before going to bed, is enjoying an active retirement. Hank continues to feel buoyed by a symbolic sense of his parents' ongoing presence as he builds a family of his own and a supportive network of friends. Emma is pursuing her career far from home with the comforting memory of her sister at her side.

We need not reduce mourning to a purely logical process in which the bereaved only accept that the other is not there. We need not live in a world of only cold facts where that which feels real holds no value, where one's most cherished relationships must be physically present in order to provide comfort and guidance. Something much more complex is afoot. Healthy mourning demands both a process of relinquishing bonds, of *absence*, while also maintaining some semblance of *presence*. I have come to think of these seemingly dichotomous measures of healthy mourning as a unified, dialectical whole, what I call *absence-and-presence*: acceptance for what has been lost alongside an ongoing and uplifting attachment to the deceased.

Problems ensue when the bereaved walk on one side of this tension while sidestepping the other. In terms of Hegelian dialectics, dichotomous thinking threatens to complicate the mourning process if affirmation of either absence or presence is taken to negate the other. Some, like Leroy, suffer from privileging the importance of accepting reality (absence) at the expense of finding no value in continuing bonds (presence). They may be too quick to nullify connections to the past and hastily arrive at a new reality without proper preparations, or they may refuse to acknowledge how helpful it can be to occasionally turn back to the memories of the deceased for warmth and guidance as they embark upon new ventures.

Others, like Sabrina, maintain continuing bonds (presence) at the expense of shirking the need to relinquish some of the past (absence) and embrace more of what follows. Negative continuing bonds abound in such cases: anxious attachments to inanimate objects that represent the dead, all-consuming preoccupations with memories of the deceased, and hesitation to pursue new relationships after a loss. Despite intentions to manage the pain of grief by holding on to the past, excessive presence only plunges the bereaved further into a state of interminable distress. Continuing bonds ultimately fail to provide any true comfort and shut down exploration of the future if not tempered with acceptance of absence.

Absence-and-presence denotes a synthesis of objective reality and the subjective experience of ongoing connection to the deceased into a meaningful whole greater than the sum of its parts. These two components of mourning complement and even enhance each other. The symbolic *presence* of continuing bonds is indicative of healthy mourning only insofar as it is a transitional experience that simultaneously accommodates the reality of *absence*. And the stark reality of death and *absence* is assuaged and made tolerable if the bereaved individual can hold the deceased's comforting *presence* in their heart and mind.

Culture and the individual's subjectivity

Each individual differs in the degree to which he or she manages to strike a healthy balance between all that mourning demands. Though it is healthy to express feelings of grief, some drown in their tears, whereas others' eyes remain a bit too dry. It is restorative to embrace life after loss, but some sprint too fast towards the future while others cower from what awaits. And as much as there is a place for continuing bonds in mourning, some live entirely in the shadow of past interactions with the dead, whereas others never allow themselves a moment to suspend reality and access the illusory comforts of felt presence.

Similarly, each culture's collective practices, values, and beliefs accentuate certain elements of the mourning process while giving less emphasis to others. Wildly eclectic grief rituals enacted from one culture to the next represent more than a scattershot of disparate ideas about how to mourn. They converge around the most common aspects of how to cope with loss in a meaningful way: painful yearning for reunion, angry protests against absence, the impulse to search for the deceased, slow and painstaking admissions of defeat in the face of reality, the compromised solution of maintaining an ongoing symbolic bond with the dead, and the psychological imperative to move forward.

The agony of grief and mourning may be ubiquitous, but its manifest expression varies greatly from one individual to the next. Cultural grief rituals provide a helpful signpost for how members of the community can embody their pain. And yet time and again those left to passively rely upon what culture provides are prone to feel that something distinctive about their subjective experience of mourning is not being voiced, drowned out in an undifferentiated choir of chants. The collective prescription often fails to alleviate what aches within one.

Those who are let down by what culture offers can opt to play a more active role in their own journey through mourning. The individual can harness creativity and design personal grief rituals that meet specific needs and affirm what was unique about the relationship they had with the deceased. Personal grief rituals can create activities through which the bereaved embody a more meaningful expression of what has been lost. They can be tailored to facilitate whichever feeling states require further venting. And they can help achieve absence-and-presence by countering whatever is impeding so that the bereaved can move forward while also maintaining a meaningful connection to those they still love. Lastly, the individual who takes the reins and guides themselves through mourning is more empowered for having articulated what the subjective experience of loss means to them, what it is they need in order to heal, and how to give oneself what they once depended upon culture to provide.

References

Ainsworth, M. D. (1963). The development of infant-mother interaction among the Ganda. In B. M. Foss (Ed.), *Determinants of infant behavior* (pp. 67–112). Wiley.

Ainsworth, M. D., & Wittig, B. A. (1969). Attachment and exploratory behavior of one-year-olds in a strange situation. In B. M. Foss (Ed.), *Determinants of infant behavior* (Vol. 4, pp. 113–136). Methuen.

Ainsworth, M. D. S., Bell, S. M., & Stayton, D. J. (1971). Individual differences in strange-situation behavior of one-year-olds. In H. R. Schaffer (Ed.), *The origins of human social relations* (pp. 17–58). Academic Press.

Ainsworth, M. D. S., Blehar, M. C., Waters, E., & Wall, S. (1978). *Patterns of attachment: A psychological study of the strange situation*. Erlbaum.

Antonucci, T. C., Akiyama, H., & Takahashi, K. (2004). Attachment and close relationships across the life span. *Attachment & Human Development, 6*(4), 353–370.

Bakermans-Kranenburg, M., & van IJzendoorn, M. (2009). The first 10,000 adult attachment interviews: Distributions of adult attachment representations in clinical and non-clinical groups. *Attachment & Human Development, 11*(3), 223–263.

Bifulco, A., Moran, P. M., Ball, C., & Bernazzani, O. (2002). Adult attachment style. I: Its relationship to clinical depression. *Social Psychiatry and Psychiatric Epidemiology, 37*, 50–59.

Blatt, S. J. (2006). A fundamental polarity in psychoanalysis: Implications for personality development, psychopathology, and the therapeutic process. *Psychoanalytic Inquiry, 26*(4), 494–520.

Bonanno, G., & Kaltman, S. (2001). The varieties of grief experience. *Clinical Psychology Review, 21*, 705–734.

Boorstin, D. J. (1983). *The discoverers: A history of man's search to know his world and himself.* Random House.

Bowlby, J. (1963). Pathological mourning and childhood mourning. *Journal of the American Psychoanalytic Association, 11*, 500–541.

Bowlby, J. (1973). *Attachment and loss: Vol. 2. Separation: Anxiety and anger*. Basic Books.

Bowlby, J. (1980). *Attachment and loss: Vol. 3. Loss: Sadness and depression*. Basic Books.

Field, N. (2006). Unresolved grief and continuing bonds: An attachment perspective. *Death Studies, 30*, 739–756.

Fraley, R. C., & Bonanno, G. A. (2004). Attachment and loss: A test of three competing models on the association between attachment-related avoidance and adaptation to bereavement. *Personality and Social Psychology Bulletin, 30*, 878–890.

Freud, S. (1917). Mourning and melancholia. *Standard Edition, 14*, 243–258. Hogarth Press.

Gorer, G. (1965). *Death, grief, and mourning*. Doubleday.

Green, B. L., Furrer, C., & McAllister, C. (2007). How do relationships support parenting? Effects of attachment style and social support on parenting behavior in an at-risk population. *American Journal of Community Psychology, 40*, 96–108.

Hill-Soderlund, A. L., Mills-Koonce, W. R., Propper, C., Calkins, S. D., Granger, D. A., & Moore, G. A. (2008). Parasympathetic and sympathetic responses to the strange situation in infants and mothers from avoidant and securely attached dyads. *Developmental Psychobiology, 50*(4), 361–376.

Jacobsen, T., & Hoffman, V. (1997). Children's attachment representations: Longitudinal relations to school behavior and academic competency in middle childhood and adolescence. *Developmental Psychology, 33*, 703–710.

Klass, D., Silverman, P., & Nickman, S. (1996). *Continuing bonds: New understandings of grief.* Taylor & Francis.

Kobak, R. R., Cole, H. E., Ferenz-Gillies, R., Flemming, W. S., & Gamble, W. (1993). Attachment and emotional regulation during mother-teen problem-solving. A control theory analysis. *Child Development, 64*, 231–245.

Kotler, T., Buzwell, S., Romeo, Y., & Bowland, J. (1994). Avoidant attachment as a risk factor for health. *The British Journal of Medical Psychology, 67*(3), 237–245.

Larose, S., & Bernier, A. (2001). Social support processes: Mediators of attachment state of mind and adjustment in late adolescence. *Attachment and Human Development, 3*, 96–120.

Mahler, M. S. (1971). A study of the separation-individuation process: And its possible application to borderline phenomena in the psychoanalytic situation. *The Psychoanalytic Study of the Child, 26*, 403–424.

Mahler, M. S., Pine, F., & Bergman, A. (1975). *The psychological birth of the human infant.* Basic Books.
Mancini, A. D., & Bonanno, G. A. (2012). The persistence of attachment: Complicated grief, threat, and reaction times to the deceased's name. *Journal of Affective Disorders, 139,* 256–263.
Meier, A. M., Carr, D. R., Currier, J. M., & Neimeyer, R. A. (2013). Attachment anxiety and avoidance in coping with bereavement: Two studies. *Journal of Social and Clinical Psychology, 32,* 315–334.
Mikulincer, M., Gillath, O., & Shaver, P. R. (2002). Activation of the attachment system in adulthood: Threat-related primes increase the accessibility of mental representations of attachment figures. *Journal of Personality and Social Psychology, 83,* 881–895.
Piaget, J. (1954). *The construction of reality in the child.* Basic Books.
Shuchter, S. R., & Zisook, S. (1986). Treatment of spousal bereavement: A multidimensional approach. *Psychiatric Annals, 16*(5), 295–305.
Sroufe, L. A., & Waters, E. (1977). Heart rate as a convergent measure in clinical and developmental research. *Merrill-Palmer Quarterly, 23*(1), 3–27.
Stroebe, M., & Schut, H. (1999). The dual process model of coping with bereavement: Rationale and description. *Death Studies, 23,* 197–224.
Stroebe, M., & Schut, H. (2010). The dual process model: A decade on. *OMEGA – Journal of Death and Dying, 61,* 273–291.
Stroebe, M., Schut, H., & Stroebe, W. (2005). Attachment in coping with bereavement: A theoretical integration. *Review of General Psychology, 9,* 48–66.
Volkan, V. D. (1972). The linking objects of pathological mourners. *Archives of General Psychiatry, 27*(2), 215–221.
Wallin, D. J. (2007). *Attachment in psychotherapy.* Guilford Press.
Waters, E., Merrick, S., Treboux, D., Crowell, J., & Albersheim, L. (2000). Attachment security in infancy and early adulthood: A twenty-year longitudinal study. *Child Development, 71,* 684–689.
Wijngaards-de Meij, L., Stroebe, M., Schut, H., Stroebe, W., Van den Bout, J., van der Heijden, P. G., & Dijkstra, I. (2007). Patterns of attachment and parents' adjustment to the death of their child. *Personality and Social Psychology Bulletin, 33,* 537–548.
Winnicott, D. W. (1953). Transitional objects and transitional phenomena – A study of the first not-me possession. *The International Journal of Psychoanalysis, 34,* 89–97.
Winnicott, D. W. (1960). The theory of the parent-infant relationship. *The International Journal of Psychoanalysis, 41,* 585–595.
Worden, J. W. (2008). *Grief counseling and grief therapy: A handbook for the mental health practitioner* (4th ed.). Springer Publishing Company.

Chapter 3

Designing personal grief rituals

In the chapters that follow, we will become acquainted with a host of individuals who created a personal grief ritual that helped them overcome suffering and mourn with greater meaning: a young woman who went searching for her father near his old workbench in the garage despite knowing he was no longer there; a middle-aged man who released purple balloons into the air to bid farewell to his lifelong friend; a daughter who decided to wear a bright and spirited dress to display the joy she managed to hold on to after her mother's death; a mother who directed her anger towards an empty chair as if her deceased son were sitting in it; a young man who attended a theater production alongside the imagined company of his sister just like they did in childhood; a bereaved husband who walked wooded paths and nature reserves his wife never had the chance to explore before her sudden death; and a woman who liberated herself from her ex-husband's specter by setting his clothes ablaze and basking in the hot flames. But before we consider how they each managed to carve their own unique path through mourning, we must ask ourselves: *Why might the bereaved turn away from what culture provides them in mourning?*

Why cultural rituals fail the individual

Across epochs of time, and in every corner of the world, culture has resorted to rituals to facilitate grief and mourning. A survey of their varied forms is an awe-inspiring testament to humanity's immense potential for creativity, its great diversity of belief systems regarding death, and its ability to give form to the nebulous pangs of loss through a wide range of symbols and behaviors. But the kaleidoscopic variations between one individual's subjective experience of loss and the next cast doubt on any culture being able to accommodate all its members. Metcalf and Huntington (1991) stated:

> Whatever mental adjustments the individual needs to make in the face of death he or she must accomplish as best as he or she can through or around such rituals as society provides. No doubt the rites frequently aid

DOI: 10.4324/9781351204873-3

> adjustment. But we have no reason to believe that they do not obstruct it with equal frequency.
>
> (p. 62)

Collective traditions thwart the individual in myriad ways. For starters, institutionalized grief rituals are prone to stifle one's need for authentic emotional expression. Wouters (2002) has used the phrase *regime of silence* to note the problem of fixed and uniform grief rituals offering a *we-feeling* of connectedness at the expense of subordinating *I-feelings*. This echoes Durkheim's observations about how rituals systematically tamp down the emotional timbre of certain feelings. In pursuit of social cohesion, the group must narrow its expressions of grief and mourning and, in doing so, disenfranchise the profane interests of the individual. Buddhists and the Bara of Madagascar alike forbid extensive displays of sadness amid mourning, whereas bereaved individuals in Hawaii, a tribe of Australian Aboriginals, or certain Arab sects are compelled to manifest shows of grief regardless of what they are actually feeling.

Assigned emotional responses are regularly steeped in a culture's rigid gender roles, with women typically expected to express grief while men are to remain stoic. This is a grave disservice to both parties, as available options for how to feel in mourning are cleaved off. An otherwise-complex array of potential grief reactions is bifurcated and projected into a passive, effected female stance and a complementary active male stance which resists any pull to emote. In the times of ancient Greece, female singers were hired to perform theatrical funeral dirges that expressed heart-aching lamentations in honor of the dead. Emotionally evocative by design, only the females were permitted to weep, while men were prohibited from exhibiting any semblance of grief (Alexiou, 1974; Johnston, 1999).

The Nyakyusa people of Tanzania and Malawi are also subjected to gender-based restraints on emotional expression. Men are only permitted to cry once before participating in a dancing ceremony. Both women and men will engage in seductive and amorous play throughout their funerary events, but it is primarily the men who embody sexual vitality and strength through energetic dancing so as to fortify courage among mourners and help them tolerate grief. Women, however, are expected to wail and remain in a state of distress within the home where the corpse is temporarily stored until burial. Thus, men are cast into an active role that conveys strength, while the women, relegated to the confines of the home and in proximity to the deceased, embody fear (Wilson, 1939). Simone de'Beauvoir is turning in her grave!

Though continuing bonds prove to be a meaningful and potentially helpful way to cope with loss, many find themselves immersed within a culture whose customs discourage any such ongoing connections to the dead. Consider the prevalence of scientific reductionism in the Western world. Embracing the stark reality of absence and adapting to life without the deceased are seen as the highest measures of healthy mourning. Enlightenment values of reason and skepticism are privileged over more subjective perceptions of reality, and in dealing with the problem of mourning, this stoic attitude is either indifferent to or outright rejects the utility of felt presence in mourning and grief rituals. Conversely, in Japan, Mexico, and among the Tana Torajans of Indonesia, custom implores the bereaved to interact with the deceased, and it may very well be that select individuals would rather detach themselves from the dead, especially if the relationship was an unhealthy one while they were still alive.

The individual may encounter a conflict between the length of time their culture prescribes for mourning and their own ideal pace. This is particularly relevant to the liminal phase of mourning. Van Gennep (1960) observed that grief rituals exist within a framework of beliefs about how the deceased's soul is *betwixt and between* the processes of separating from life and arriving at the soul's final destination. Similarly, any given culture's customs dictate how long the bereaved are to exist within such an intermediary phase of transition through mourning: Surviving community members are neither completely separated from ties to the deceased, nor are they completely reincorporated back into life. But the timeline afforded to journey through liminality can range from three days to seven years. Consider the individual struggling with incessant expressions of grief and all-consuming continuing bonds; a protracted stay within liminality would only aggravate excessive loss-oriented stress and drag out a chronic pattern of mourning further. An inverted mismatch between society and the individual is no better. For those prone to hastily relinquish bonds and move on without processing grief, an abbreviated liminal phase would collude with psychological defenses of avoidance and increase the likelihood of a disproportionate amount of restoration-oriented stress and a delayed course of mourning.

The high potential for incompatibility between culture and the individual is undeniable. A certain proportion of bereaved members within the community are destined to fall between the cracks and find themselves wedged into a culture whose one-size-fits-all grief rituals are not in harmony with their subjective experience of loss and what they need in order to mourn. Consider the ways in which collective rituals and customs may have thwarted Mandy, Hank, or Emma. Mandy needed to hold close to the love of her life as she moved into retirement, and so she developed a personal grief ritual in which she spoke with him and addressed him by name every night. Now imagine Mandy immersed within a culture who, akin to the Japanese ritual of *kaimyo* (Swarts, 2001), discouraged her from uttering his name before falling asleep. Hank found it beneficial to visit his parents' favorite haunts and comb through albums of family photos whenever he needed to vent feelings of sadness for his loss. But what if Hank were a member of a tribe whose rituals prohibited any ongoing expression of grief and only allowed him, a man, to embody courage? Emma developed a personal grief ritual in which she embarked upon new journeys across the world to places her sister would have liked to visit. Any such drive to relish in novel and meaningful sojourns would have been quashed if one were pressured to take part in a joyless, year-long state of compulsory mourning.

Aside from conflicts between collective practices and the individual's psychological needs, many simply will not have immediate access to rituals. Firstly, grief rituals prove to be expensive affairs. The Toraja peoples of Tana Toraja work hard to accumulate wealth to fund elaborate and celebratory ceremonies. Surviving family members will sometimes require many years to reserve sufficient funds to ensure that the ceremony appropriately honors the deceased in a manner that is commensurate with the family member's status. The value of the deceased's life is put on display for the community to acknowledge, not unlike the reading of eulogies in other cultures (Budiman, 2013). Even in Haiti, a country whose development has been chronically hindered by financial crisis, more affluent families prefer to inter loved ones in aboveground tombs rather than burying the dead underground (Huggins & Hinkson, 2019). Whether in America, Indonesia, or Haiti, financial resources and socioeconomic status give privileged access to elaborate ceremonies, and a lack of money often limits a family's ability to express the depths of their grief in a fashion that is most meaningful to them. Some individuals are not able to attend simply because they can afford neither a plane ticket nor the loss of income they would endure upon taking time off from work.

The circumstances of when and how a traditional ritual is performed may be what chokes off access to some. In the Sanyuan Village of China, many grief rituals are performed prior to the moment of death. A crucial moment comes immediately before the dying family member passes away, at which point kin will gather around and bid farewell, thus releasing the deceased's soul from this world. It is not uncommon for family members who live far away to be incapable of returning to the village in time to say goodbye (Birx, 2006). In other cultures, tradition determines that only a select member or two of the family be assigned to participate in important rites. It is customary in Hindu grief rituals that the eldest son use a lighted torch to ignite the funeral pyre of a deceased parent; all other kin are left to watch passively with limited opportunity to enact any part of their grief (Laungani, 1997).

Consider the plight of minorities, removed from their country of origin, who cannot act out meaningful rituals in a foreign land. Distance from important geographical locations may be enough to hinder their performance. At other times, one group's values and beliefs are in conflict with those of the dominant culture. Immigrants regularly find themselves under pressure to conform with and adopt the predominant practices of the host culture, including any local laws and regulations which would impede upon traditional customs. Laungani (1997), speaking of the difficulties Hindus face when attempting to conduct grief rituals in Britain, states:

> The Ganges does not flow through Behtnal Green, the law does not permit bodies to be paraded through the streets without a coffin and burned on public pyres, and Western business customs do not allow a son to take twelve days off work in order to fulfill his obligations to a dead father. (pg. 67)

Even within one's home country, traditions fall out of practice or may be unavailable during a stretch of time. Many cultures have long valued direct contact with the body of the deceased, but growing health concerns stemming from improper handling of corpses have resulted in many having to abandon long-standing customs. In Madagascar, an outbreak of the bubonic plague in 2017 may have sounded the death knell for their famadihana rituals, as authorities began discouraging communities from unearthing the dead. And various tribes around the world who once used ritualistic endocannibalism as a meaningful act of mourning have since abandoned the practice. Even as this book is being completed in the year 2021, the COVID-19 pandemic continues to place limits on large social gatherings. In an effort to stave off further spread of the virus, bereaved family members have had to opt for small gatherings or virtual funerals through the internet, a cold and impersonal experience that has proven to be unsatisfying for many.

Lastly, many problems with limited access to cultural rituals can be attributed to an increasingly nomadic society and subsequent loss of community. A centralized community of people with whom one shares beliefs and values has been the cornerstone of collective rituals throughout human history. But as the individual is more regularly displaced in pursuit of education, career, and a life separate from their family of origin, the bereaved have no choice but to mourn in isolation apart from familiar practices and from those who had also known the deceased. Furthermore, per Wouters' notion of the *regime of silence*, those living in highly individualistic cultures often find that the community in which they are embedded has gone quiet in response to loss. Mourning, it seems, has vanished from public life in the Western world, diminishing opportunities to find public recognition of grief feelings or to observe others modeling how to mourn.

Wouters (2002) has described the modern-day bereaved individual as being caught in a *tug of war*, torn between the *we ideals* of institutionalized social obligations whose prescribed customs ensure solidarity amid grief, and the *I ideals* of one's own idiosyncratic impulses and personal feelings that align them with a truer course of mourning. But this balancing act has, for many, begun to tilt in favor of individualism. Numerous authors over the past three decades have commented on how the late twentieth century ushered in erosion of trust in the authority of traditions, growing dissatisfaction with institutionalized grief rituals, and a breakdown of any shared sense of meaning around death (Bolton & Camp, 1987; Fulton, 1988; Walter, 1996). Such skepticism has yielded increased interest in alternative means of interpreting the world and coping with human experiences, including the inevitability of death and the subjective experience of loss. The entire experience of mourning is slowly shifting away from rigid, sometimes-dogmatic formalities and more towards processes carried out in private, in convenience, and with deeper personal meaning.

The benefits of personal grief rituals

When collective rituals thwart one's ability to mourn, and when broad societal change is too daunting, personal grief rituals present a viable alternative. Therese Rando (1985) made an early push for more individualized solutions, saying, "the judicious creation of rituals in the therapy of the bereaved offers uniquely efficacious methods of addressing 'grief work' and constitutes a potentially powerful adjunct to traditional forms of counseling and psychotherapy" (p. 236). A wave of scholars from the fields of psychology and sociology has since echoed Rando's recommendation for the development of rituals that meet an individual's specific needs when formal institutions are not equipped to accommodate them (Lofland, 1985; Grimes, 2004; Platvoet, 1995; Wojtkowiak et al., 2021; Wouters, 2002). Bereaved individuals are taking the cue and increasingly embracing the benefits of more personalized approaches to mourning, whether as an adjunct to cultural traditions or an outright replacement. They are also beginning to appreciate that personal grief rituals can facilitate a healthier and more meaningful experience than those steeped in custom (Schachter & Finneran, 2013).

One of the greatest benefits of personal grief rituals is that they can be *tailored to meet the individual's unique psychological needs while in mourning* (Fiese et al., 2002; Romanoff & Terenzio, 1998). Too often, scholarly theories put forth rigid prescriptions for mourning that pursue the impossible goal of finding a uniform approach that works for all; these theories only perpetuate an ugly schism between recommendations of old, as if they no longer hold any value for anyone, and the new, shiny, and improved model. Rather, the correct model for how to mourn varies greatly from one individual to the next. What one person requires in order to cope with a loss hinges upon both long-standing issues, such as temperament and attachment style and the relationship they had with the deceased, and more immediate factors, such as the current experience of grief and the degree to which efforts to cope thus far are helping. It is also imperative that the bereaved walk a path that guides them through whichever facets of mourning are obstructed. The following questions, each of which corresponds to one component of

William Worden's (2008) task model, should be considered prior to designing a personal grief ritual:

- To what degree would it be helpful to confront the reality of physical absence and relinquish ties?
- What does grief genuinely feel like for the bereaved, and which emotions require greater expression? Which emotions need only limited expression?
- Might the individual benefit from enacting behaviors that facilitate forward movement and adaptation to life without the deceased, beyond the ambiguity of liminality, or is further reflection upon the past warranted?
- Would the bereaved find comfort in establishing continuing bonds with the deceased and basking in their illusory presence, or would it be better to establish further distance from the dead?

Cultural rituals appeal to a broad and diffuse set of beliefs about what the deceased had meant to the community as a whole. Personal grief rituals, on the other hand, help articulate what the deceased meant to the individual and enact how they wish to move forward while holding on or letting go of certain elements of that particular relationship. Coleman and Neimeyer (2010) have stressed the importance of meaning-making as a crucial component of the mourning process and how early successes in finding meaning predict overall well-being years after a loss. From this perspective, a personalized approach can help the bereaved affirm previous beliefs about the deceased or formulate something anew by incorporating novel thoughts, symbols, and behaviors into a revised understanding of what their loss means to them.

One of the more therapeutic properties of all grief rituals is their fixed and predictable structure and that benefit is derived from traditional customs and personal grief rituals all the same (Reeves, 2011). The course of mourning is an uneven terrain marked by stretches of calm that alternate with unexpected bumps in the road: intrusive emotional pain, unforeseen confrontations with the reality of loss that interrupt one's focus, and difficult adjustments that must be made on the fly. Ritual enactment, on the other hand, consists of predetermined sequences of behavior and a compartmentalized, time-limited framework. Its circumscribed activity takes place in a specific location with a clear beginning and end. This spatiotemporal foundation serves as the ideal container for otherwise-diffuse bouts of grief. Within the confines of a ritual's structure, the bereaved can validate their loss, separate from the deceased (Van der Hart & Ebbers, 1981), and express feelings free from concerns of being flooded with grief at inopportune times (Romanoff & Terenzio, 1998).

Ongoing research confirms the value of delimiting time to let out grief and then draw it to a close. The dual process model (DPM) of coping with bereavement has long suggested that the bereaved benefit from taking breaks from the *grief work* of loss-oriented stress and oscillating towards equally important restoration-oriented stresses, eventually oscillating back to grief work again in due time (Stroebe & Schut, 1999). However, recent advancements in this body of research have paid greater attention to the problem of stress *overload* in the mourning process (Stroebe & Schut, 2016). It has since been recommended that the bereaved take breaks from coping with loss and bereavement altogether so they can stave off burnout and restore energy before returning once more to such a demanding undertaking. From this perspective, personal grief rituals facilitate healthy mourning by providing the individual a structure that demarcates time and space for active coping and subsequent respite upon its completion. And the individual can return to the ritual as many times as he or she needs.

Designing and participating in unique ritualistic behaviors also allows the bereaved to exercise a semblance of control over the otherwise-chaotic experience of mourning (Castle & Phillips, 2003; Rando, 1985; Romanoff & Terenzio, 1998; Wyrostok, 1995). Research by Norton and Gino (2014) confirms that personal grief rituals bolster their actors with regained feelings of control. These activities provide a compensatory mechanism that fights against passivity and shields the bereaved from the bombardment of emotions that must otherwise be felt and sustained until the damage is done. By implementing personal grief rituals, the individual can take charge and actively do something about their grief. They can structure its timing and location in ways that are both meaningful and convenient. Cultural rituals just tell the bereaved where to show up and when.

Liberated from the constraints of tradition, the individual can harness his or her creativity to design a unique sequence of meaningful behaviors that meet their psychological needs. But as one problem is solved, another challenge emerges. Culturally prescribed behaviors and schemas about the meaning of loss may fail the individual at times, but those who strike out on their own to build something entirely new soon realize they have few tools in hand. A leaky roof may have been better than none at all. The institutions of culture may suffer from narrow systems of meaning and behavior amid mourning; nonetheless, they provide some shelter under which the bereaved can weather the storm. When cultural institutions are abandoned, it is incumbent on the frustrated individual to build novel structures in the dark and shoulder the difficult work of creating something of one's own making.

A warning about cultural misappropriation

Rather than jettison tradition altogether, there remains enormous value in tapping the collective wisdom of customs practiced around the world to inform the design of a personal grief ritual. The proverbial baby need not be thrown out with the bathwater. The bereaved individual who is disenfranchised from their own culture's practices can look elsewhere with curiosity and respect in hopes of finding something that awakens their subjective experience of loss, something that models a more meaningful expression of grief they would not be witness to otherwise. A particular culture might make room for specific emotions in mourning that the individual had been discouraged from feeling in their homeland. Observing a distant peoples' acts of ongoing connection to the deceased may give the individual license to create continuing bonds in spite of their home culture's insistence upon letting go.

But looking to other cultures for inspiration is a slippery slope, as it is always tempting to circumvent the difficult work of designing a unique ritual of one's own and simply adopt what others have already created. Cultural misappropriation becomes an ethical problem if the individual enacts another's practices wholesale and fails to acknowledge its true source, as if the ritual were one's own personal invention. Such mimicry is disrespectful and, furthermore, is likely to misrepresent the true meaning and complexity of what another culture cherishes and holds sacred.

Cultural misappropriation is more than a moral infraction; expropriating another's rituals is also a pragmatic problem that sets up the bereaved for failure. The individual, with his or her own presuppositions about death and mourning, is likely to obscure the true meaning and purpose behind what they borrow from the other, ultimately leaving them befuddled as to what they are doing. The bereaved would not likely benefit from a cursory reading of Hindu death rituals and a hasty decision to pour various vessels of water into one another as an act of mourning. Ironically, imitating an unfamiliar practice threatens to repeat the original problem that drove them to look elsewhere in the first place: numb participation in behaviors that lack genuine meaning for the participant. Cultural misappropriation of grief rituals runs the risk of leaving the bereaved no better off for having enacted something which had no personal meaning to them. Those who are too eager to borrow tools they do not know how to use are fated to build a ramshackle house.

This book implores those who are frustrated with what their culture provides to create grief rituals that are unique, personal, and of their own design. And . . . it is perfectly reasonable to look elsewhere for inspiration. Humans do not evolve separate from one another. Different peoples benefit from exchanging wisdom about how to best manage the difficult tasks of mourning. To that end, we will not only study different cultures' attempts to cope with loss but will also look to many different individuals and observe the grief rituals they intuitively created on their own. A true dialectic is to be struck between culture and the individual, where the bereaved can lean upon the tried-and-true beliefs of many while also accessing the more personal and private experience of what their loss means to them. One might not wish to replicate Hindu mourning rituals exactly as they are practiced in Nepal and India, but if the thought of carrying water or wielding fire inspires a unique and personally meaningful expression of mourning, there is no shame in taking a nod from those who came before.

Righting the ship: Creating personal grief rituals in psychotherapy

Laungani (1997) stated, "The priest sees death as a transition for the dead whereas the psychotherapist sees it as a transition for the bereaved" (p. 235). Psychotherapists have long argued for grief rituals to be woven into standard psychotherapeutic practices (Al-Krenawi, 1999; Doka, 2012; Romanoff & Terenzio, 1998; Van der Hart, 1983). Talk therapy, as it were, too often privileges language above all else. Its method values stillness. Sitting motionless and talking ad nauseum about loss and mourning leave the bereaved frustrated, yearning to actively do something. Participation within rituals augments traditional psychotherapeutic interventions with the opportunity to be more actively engaged in mourning and counter the passive experience of grief happening to the bereaved. Palazzoli et al. (1978) observed that physical enactment of emotions predicts positive change more than verbalization, and Reeves (2011) has echoed the importance of full mind-body engagement during the enactment of rituals.

The design of a personal grief ritual must ascertain what is needed in order to facilitate a healthy and meaningful passage through mourning. This is a perplexing task filled with hypotheses that seem to contradict one another. Might the bereaved benefit from greater confrontation with the reality of loss, or are they already bombarded with excessive reminders of absence? Should rituals foster ongoing felt presence and continuing bonds that provide safe shelter from the emptiness of grief, or is it more warranted to cast off attachments to past ties? Is greater emotional expression in order, or should it be limited and contained? Would the bereaved be well-advised to turn towards memories of the past, or would it be better to orient oneself more towards future endeavors?

A kernel of truth resides in each of these polarized possibilities. Healthy mourning amounts to a balancing act that reconciles opposing forces of absence-and-presence: grief-laden expressions of protest alternating with retreat from emotional overload, remembrances that pull for reflections on the past and a simultaneous push to point one's feet towards new ventures, acceptance for the absence of what has been lost alongside ongoing attachment to the deceased. Most bereaved individuals maintain equilibrium; they resort to grief rituals merely as a way to imbue greater meaning into the mourning process. Others, however, succumb to a complicated course of bereavement largely because *their subjective experience of loss and mourning sets them off-kilter*.

A self-directed approach to designing personal grief rituals presupposes that the individual's proclivities about how to mourn are commensurate with what will, in fact, usher in health. But the same faulty instincts that take some down a painful path of grief may inspire the pursuit of activities that mislead them further and exacerbate suffering and dysfunction along the way. Their compass fails to point towards true north. Some, like Leroy, falsely believe that burying seemingly messy and useless emotions as soon as possible is the best course of action, whereas others, like Sabrina, are stuck because they feel that the pinnacle of effective mourning entails an interminable walk down memory lane. In such cases, personal grief rituals must be designed to recalibrate what has led the individual astray and help to circumvent that which has obstructed their journey thus far.

Those embroiled in complicated bereavement will benefit from the assistance of a professional to right the ship and lay out a corrective course that counters imbalances. As Rabkin (1977) remarked, "Patients attempt to master their problems with a strategy which, because it is unsuccessful, the therapist changes" (p. 5). The reticent individual suffering from masked grief will benefit from a ritual that elicits more emotion, whereas the person mired in chronic grief will be aided by behaviors that nudge them ever so slightly away from the past. A ritual's structure can bracket off time and space to intentionally engage in healing activities that do not necessarily come naturally to the individual.

There is no shortage of irony in retreating from the frustrations of what one source of authority, culture, has prescribed only to seek refuge in what a psychotherapist, and the field of psychology as a whole, might recommend. Out of the frying pan and into the fire, the schism between a collective will and personal needs threatens to widen further. But the individual can coexist in a creative and collaborative relationship with others. The dyad of therapist and bereaved client works together as a more ideal collective in which the professional shines a light in the direction that leads to the healthiest course while still enlisting the client's active participation in creating and enacting meaningful expressions of grief and mourning along the way.

Bereaved clients stand to gain the most from working with their therapists to develop personal grief rituals that are unique and personally meaningful to them. Wyrostok (1995) observed that rituals designed for a particular client will have certain elements that make it outright inappropriate or irrelevant for others. What is profound for one is a vapid and empty gesture for another. And so the ritual's design must be informed by an excavation of one's personal history, an unearthing of true feelings about the deceased, and the discovery of meaningful activities and symbols tied to their subjective experience of the loss.

Yes, it is a great mass of variables to consider, and the process of two people working together to design something anew can undoubtedly be trying. Nonetheless, a collaborative approach is far superior to a therapist simply assigning generic rituals for the bereaved to perform. It is all too common for professionals to hastily advise writing a letter to the deceased, spreading ashes into a body of water, or placing a framed picture within the home without taking time to elicit the client's thoughts or contributions. The bereaved often seek out professional help in retreat from pressures to parrot what somebody else had prescribed. The low-hanging fruit of prepackaged rituals would only invite the same stale ceremonialism they ran from in the first place. To design a unique and personally meaningful grief ritual that meets the individual's specific needs and is suited to their subjective experience of loss is a worthwhile challenge and one that has proven to be efficacious even in cases of prolonged grief (Wojtkowiak et al., 2021).

Lastly, no matter how much the professional guides the process, they should insist that the client actively participate in creating his or her own personal grief rituals. In time, what began as a joint effort in creativity galvanizes the bereaved to eventually go it alone when needed or desired, exhibiting a greater capacity to provide for themselves whatever assistance and guidance they had initially relied upon the therapist for. Not unlike the child equipped with an internal representation of the attachment figure who can venture farther away, so too can the bereaved client internalize the therapeutic relationship and steady himself on two feet to walk forward, ever deeper into his own personal journey through loss, grief, and mourning.

Assessment: Ascertaining excess and deficiency

Mourning demands so much from those afflicted by loss: flexibility in coping with loss-oriented stress and restoration-oriented stress, the patience to confront and steadily absorb the reality of absence, healthy emotional expression, adaptations to life without the deceased, maintenance of continuing bonds. These measures of healthy mourning must be tended to in balance with one another, and it appears that long-standing elements of personality play a critical role in determining the likelihood that a state of equilibrium, of absence-and-presence, is maintained. Certain character traits and behavioral tendencies provide fortification against the harsh onslaught of mourning, while others raise the odds of an imbalanced and weakened defense. For instance, one's general coping style either gravitates towards active strategies that approach the strains of loss head-on or passive strategies that evade uncomfortable thoughts and feelings.

Attachment style is one such component of personality that has been shown to be predictive of the course that mourning takes (Schenck et al., 2016). And it should come as no surprise that those with a secure attachment style are most likely to traverse mourning unscathed. Their internal working model (IWM) suggests that a need to emote feelings of grief is essentially good and likely to be helpful, and so this occurs free of inhibition. He or she turns to others for comfort. On a symbolic level, object constancy allows the bereaved to seek out memories of the deceased and continuing bonds as meaningful representations of the deceased that provide ongoing comfort. Lastly, the individual with secure attachment exhibits a propensity for exploration amid the mourning process; they are willing to break away from ties to the past and engage with novel situations and relationships after a loss because they fully trust that they can return to fond recollections as needed.

Still, the specific circumstances of a loss may provoke uncharacteristic reactions and struggles. An individual's unique relationship with the deceased can determine the course of mourning, as one death is bound up with markedly different meaning and emotional responses than another. Those who typically utilize an active coping style and embody a secure attachment style may nonetheless succumb to a particularly stressful loss and exhibit unhealthy coping typically associated with insecure attachment, such as heightened or constrained emotional expression. Lastly, cultural rituals that the bereaved are exposed to can either facilitate healthy mourning or be a hindrance regardless of long-standing personality traits.

Personal grief rituals can certainly provide auxiliary support to those whose natural dispositions have already cleared a healthy and balanced path through mourning. They may even augment the benefits that cultural rituals have provided: additional time to express emotions, further opportunities to say goodbye to the deceased, more avenues towards continuing bonds. But for those struggling to cope with loss, a personalized approach becomes necessary.

Each measure of healthy mourning described above is highly variable from one individual to the next, and *it is imperative to assess the degree to which one is struggling with an excess or deficiency of what is needed*. The bereaved individual's pains and inhibitions point to specific cracks in the dam that threaten to buckle under the pressure of bereavement. In order to ensure that the right spots are being patched up through the design of a personal grief ritual, we must now hark back to our study of the subjective experience of loss to lay out areas of inquiry that will help gauge which factors are complicating the mourning process.

Absence – acceptance and forward movement

Worden's task model, discussed in Chapter 1, is a helpful framework for sorting out which facets of mourning are being tended to, which have been neglected, and which are perhaps being overindulged. Task I denotes the necessity of accepting the reality of a loss and facing the many painful reminders of what is gone. One may be able to utter rote acknowledgments that death has occurred, but all parties helping to design a meaningful ritual should consider the possibility that the bereaved is not fully embracing the grim actualities of loss and absence. A variety of behaviors suggests deficient confrontation with reality. Bedrooms are preserved as shrines to the past. Clothes remain hung in the closet, ready for regular use. Vacant properties are perpetually left off the marketplace. Grave sites continue to be neglected as well-intended visitations and plans to adorn the headstone with flowers are repeatedly postponed. It is equally important to determine *if loss is confronted in excess*, leaving the bereaved overwhelmed by sorrowful reminiscences and upsetting encounters with the stark reality of death, like a wide-eyed deer blinded by headlights, unable to proceed forward.

Task III highlights how adaptive it is to search for new connections and experiences after a loss, ultimately building upon exploratory behaviors that were hopefully cultivated in the formative years of childhood. Trust in the ongoing availability of what is familiar is in harmonious balance with trust in one's efficacy to master the unfamiliar. Some, however, are not oriented enough towards exploring life after a loss. Any attempts to adjust to the world are stilted or avoided altogether, often as a result of self-doubt. All that lies ahead waits patiently, but the individual remains bogged down in the past, procrastinates, and never shows up. Conversely, some err towards excessive adjustment to life without the deceased. The bereaved individual masquerades as having quickly adapted, but a hasty focus on new life is often fueled by a fearful aversion to memory even as ghosts follow close behind and whisper in their ear.

Presence – continuing bonds

The tasks of mourning that entail coping with absence exist in concert with those that cultivate a degree of felt presence or, according to Task IV in William Worden's model, an enduring connection with the deceased. And therein lies the value of *absence-and-presence* as a marker of healthy mourning: Illusory experiences of an ongoing connection to the deceased are managed not in spite of the truth but alongside confrontations with the reality of loss. Here, too, the bereaved can suffer from insufficient or from excessive presence, and personal grief rituals can be designed to either promote continuing bonds or, when necessary, loosen ties.

Each individual, per their IWM, harbors beliefs about whether or not to seek out others to manage emotional upset. These attitudes must be excavated and examined prior to the design of a personal grief ritual, not only because they illuminate the degree to which the bereaved is likely to use surviving relationships to cope with grief, but also because they reveal whether or not they are leaning on the abstractions of continuing bonds for comfort. The following questions can be used to delve into this further: *Has it been helpful to turn to others for emotional support? Do you recall any fond memories of (the person you lost)? Do you ever let yourself have imaginary conversations with him/her? Do you feel an ongoing sense connection or closeness in any meaningful way?* During an intake appointment, I always ask a question or two about the relationship the bereaved had with the deceased prior to death, not only because I want to learn about the quality of the attachment, but also because I want to see how well they can access memories of the attachment figure.

A personal grief ritual may be charged with no greater task than to enact an already-existing connection to the deceased to ease the bite of grief and mourning further. Some, however, are pained by a lack of continuing bonds and a great sense of emptiness. Deficiency in presence is often due to a dismissing attachment style and an IWM that instinctively flinches at the idea of remaining close. The possibility of seeking out others has come to evoke such futility that any impulse to rediscover the deceased, even within the mind, is deactivated. Continuing bonds offer no soothing because there quite simply is no internal mental representation of the dead to which one can turn.

It is also possible for continuing bonds to be excessive. Mourning can be encumbered by an unrelenting connection to the dead. Otherwise, healthy *transitional experiences* that straddle the fence between reality and fantasy collapse into maladaptive *linking experiences* if an ongoing sense of presence is not appreciated for the illusion that it is. The most notable feature of this malady, often found in those with a preoccupied attachment style, involves constant monitoring of whatever abstract ties the bereaved has held on to. The individual is preoccupied with efforts to conjure up the other's felt presence, seemingly tethered to ties from the past they hope to preserve exactly as they were. Any impulse to explore and adapt to life beyond mourning is sacrificed in order to remain in vigil. Forward movement, they fear, will carry them too far away from past bonds. Those afflicted with such anxiety do not trust that memories and felt presence will remain in sight and within reach should they step away for a moment, like a sailor fixing his gaze on the shoreline, terrified to find that it grows ever smaller as the boat drifts out into the sea.

Whether an assessment reveals that more or less continuing bonds are in order, it is helpful to take inventory of any behaviors or inanimate objects that provide a meaningful connection to the lost relationship: activities they once enjoyed doing together, significant objects and symbols that represent a unique bond, even the deceased's characteristic behaviors and attitudes that the bereaved might be inclined to emulate. Symbolic items and activities can then be incorporated meaningfully into the creation of a personal grief ritual, whether the symbolic connection is amplified and drawn near in the process or minimized and ultimately discarded.

Lastly, it is important to note that personal grief rituals aiming to establish the correct balance of presence are helpful only insofar as they are preserving some degree of comfort or guidance associated with the deceased. Continuing bonds can be altogether problematic if they shackle the bereaved to negative aspects of a departed relationship. A thorough assessment should consider the possibility that minimal continuing bonds are an adaptive response to loss when there was little of meaning within the relationship to hold on to. And in those instances where the relationship was outright unhealthy, even abusive, continuing bonds are best cleaved off wholesale. For those individuals haunted by echoes of a harmful relationship, the healthiest degree of presence is none.

Emotional expression – containment and expansion

Task II of Worden's model addresses how important it is to process and express a variety of difficult feelings about loss without drowning in tears or boiling over in angry fits of protest. But many fall short of hitting this ideal.

It is crucial to determine if grief is pouring out in excess and unabated over time or if an insufficient outlet leaves emotions choked off and seeping out in unconscious, wordless forms that wreak havoc on one's relationships, work life, and physical health. The following questions can prove helpful in understanding this matter: *"How often do you cry since your father died?" "What kind of emotions have you been feeling about the loss?" "Has it felt helpful to express your feelings?"*

Too many bereaved individuals attempt to hide from grief. This is often the case for those who exhibit a dismissing attachment style, whose IWM leads them to believe that emotional expression will only invite upset that yields no resolution of pain. Others, such as those with a preoccupied attachment style, err more towards accentuating emotional distress that only upsets them further and affords no catharsis.

It is imperative that all parties involved in the creation of a personal grief ritual gauge the specific feelings which color the individual's subjective experience of loss. Furthermore, the meaning behind certain emotions is often less obvious than what initially meets the eye. Seemingly run-of-the-mill sadness can point specifically to regret for having squandered opportunities to build a meaningful relationship while there was still a chance; thus, in lieu of there having been a significant relationship to lose, a melancholic mood represents sadness for the loss of further time to develop a relationship worth mourning. Guilt is often at the forefront of what the bereaved is feeling, and however quick we are to assume that personal responsibility for the other's death is unfounded, the bereaved may need to work through some semblance of genuine culpability. Anger may be directed more towards the deceased and less about the deceased having died if the relationship was saturated with resentment and other hard feelings that the bereaved can no longer work out directly with their appropriate target. Rather than design rituals that simply elicit or contain a diffuse outpouring of emotion, healthy mourning is more likely to unfold if the personal meaning behind tears, or a smile, or a clenched fist is made conscious in the process.

DPM oscillations – loss- and restoration-oriented stress

Extensive research on the dual process model (DPM) of coping with bereavement asserts that the bereaved fare better if they oscillate back and forth between managing different stresses. A healthy degree of loss-oriented stress is apparent in the individual's ability to reflect upon the past and process grief about the loss of a relationship. Restoration-oriented stress is being managed well if grief work can be temporarily avoided in order to deal with situational stresses following the loss. Balance between the two is essential.

Failure to balance these stresses manifests in notably different complications that must be eased with more fluid oscillations. Insufficient restoration-oriented stress leaves the bereaved mired in chronic grief and neglecting adaptation. Perseverative thoughts about the deceased bog them down in the past and lead to bungled efforts to engage in work and surviving relationships. Alternatively, insufficient loss-oriented stress finds the bereaved avoiding the need to process grief, concerning themselves only with "moving on" and adapting to a new life at a hurried pace. They often harbor negative attitudes about how reflecting on the past would only waste their time, but closer inspection reveals an aversion to the depths of pain that would be uncovered if they were to step back momentarily from present-day endeavors and talk about what they have lost.

Immediate circumstances can determine which type of stress the bereaved overemphasizes and which is neglected. For instance, excessive restoration-oriented stress is an adaptive response for those who must assume enormous responsibility after a death. Loss within a family or larger community often leaves responsibilities and roles once filled by the deceased vacant, and it is commonplace for a single bereaved individual to bear the burden of filling this *role vacuum*, necessitating that they suppress their own grief work (loss-oriented stress) to restore order for the sake of the larger system of those in mourning.

Or it may be that the specific nature of the lost relationship determines the relative balance. Numerous interpersonal dynamics can saddle the bereaved with a disproportionate amount of grief work and a strong aversion to adaptation. For example, a pattern of heightened dependence upon the attachment figure predisposes the bereaved to feeling helpless in their absence. If the bereaved individual had consulted the attachment figure about all decisions, turned to them alone every time they needed to be soothed, and leaned upon their skillset to accomplish various goals, loss leaves the survivor feeling terrifyingly unmoored as they navigate a future alone. Fear predominates as one confronts self-doubt and low trust about their own ability to do for themselves what they once relied upon the deceased to take care of. While this type of enmeshed and codependent relationship can be the product of a preoccupied attachment style, a detailed assessment of the individual's history may reveal that other losses were managed without such struggles, suggesting that there is something about the loss of *this* relationship that leaves them painfully uncertain about how to manage the stress of what comes next in life.

Liminality and sustained ambiguity

In the weeks and months following a loss, the bereaved find themselves in a rather-vague phase of mourning, betwixt and between a past they have not quite let go of and a future which they have not decidedly stepped into just yet. This is precisely what the concept of *liminality* entails: an intermediary period in which there has been neither a firm sense of separation nor transition. Anthropological observations of cultural rituals around the world suggest that liminality is a universal and inevitable phase of mourning.

Problems ensue when this appropriately ambiguous process is either prematurely terminated or prolonged indefinitely. Thus, liminality is essentially a matter of wading through time at an appropriate clip, a temporal balancing act: neither too fast nor too slow. The liminal phase of mourning is rife with analogies to those situations in life that feel awkward if too brief or if sustained for too long. Spend twenty minutes at a traffic light and you will begin to feel restless, quite literally stuck somewhere you should have gotten past in quicker fashion. Stop into your workplace for five minutes, where you usually stay for stretches of eight or more hours, and notice how uncanny it feels to leave so soon.

Just as different cultures assume a distinctive pace through liminality that hinges upon collective beliefs about death, so too does the individual carry a distinct and subjective sense of how much time is needed to fully mourn and whether or not it is progressing at a desirable speed. Some find themselves stuck within chronic grief, struggling to move forward as they remain tethered to the past for too long. Others eventually realize that they marched too quickly ahead, that they transitioned without sufficiently separating from the deceased. They sense that some element of grief was left unprocessed and continues to linger, akin to cultural beliefs about the liminality of the deceased's soul and its capacity to haunt the living until it is resolutely released from this world.

Risks and clinical contraindications

An in-depth assessment of the individual's subjective experience of loss illuminates the personal meaning behind their grief and the mourning process. It elucidates complications to be corrected and a course of mourning that could be made more meaningful and healing. A thorough assessment can also highlight those cases in which personal grief rituals run the risk of being unhelpful. Ritualized activities have powerful effects on their participants that may prove to be too difficult to manage. Evocative expressions of grief plunge the bereaved into strong emotional responses that are unbearable for some. They can thrust participants into overwhelming confrontations with loss. If designed or implemented in a haphazard manner, personal grief rituals carry the potential to cause significant distress or exacerbate psychological ailments.

Only a trained clinical psychologist, psychiatrist, or counselor should provide formal mental health diagnoses. Nonetheless, there is value in the professional and the layperson alike being thoughtful of how bereavement can be further complicated by a full-blown psychological disorder, what Worden (2008) referred to as *exaggerated grief*. In these cases, psychological treatment from a licensed professional is the priority; the development and implementation of personal grief rituals should either be postponed until the bereaved is healthier or used with extra caution as no more than an auxiliary therapeutic activity. The following represents a short list of common psychological disorders to consider.

The unrelenting dysphoria of major depressive disorder (MDD) is certainly cause for concern. Recurrent waves of sadness are a common component of healthy mourning for many individuals. However, bouts of crying are beyond the pale when they persist unabated for days on end with no reprieve and are accompanied by a host of additional symptoms. The bereaved individual suffering from MDD will likely experience a constricted range of melancholic feelings in which there is no room for joy. Relationships and goal-directed activities may be markedly difficult to enjoy. Low energy, difficulty concentrating, disruptions in appetite and sleep, and poor self-regard tend to go hand in hand with MDD as well. Lastly, and of utmost importance, the unremitting intensity of sadness may even inspire hopelessness and give rise to thoughts of self-harm or suicide. MDD can be lethal if not treated by a trained professional.

Other mood disorders, such as bipolar affective disorder (BAD), are marked more by labile mood. That is, the range of emotions is a chaotic interchange of elated euphoria within a manic episode and the crushing sadness of depression. Volatile highs spur the individual towards reckless pursuit of pleasure and excessive goal-oriented activity, all in service of denying the lows waiting on the other end of the inevitable crash. More than mere flashes of anger or bursts of energy amid grief, all of which are unremarkable features of normal bereavement, the irritability that characterizes a manic episode proves unmanageable and regularly precedes self-destructive behavior. Personal grief rituals should be careful not to stoke more of these feelings and impulses when someone is suffering from BAD, which would be akin to pouring gasoline on an open fire.

The death of a loved one heightens awareness of mortality and unease about one's own eventual nonexistence, but such discomfort can promote active contemplation of how to live a meaningful and fulfilling life with the time that remains. The loss of a valued relationship also aggravates separation anxiety, but here, too, the attachment behaviors that follow help to steadily confront the reality of absence. Anxiety is yet another common, self-corrective response to loss that may billow into a disordered state if fails to facilitate the mourning process and, instead, comes to obstruct it.

In all their forms, anxiety disorders (agoraphobia, obsessive-compulsive disorder, phobias) following a loss are marked by efforts to avoid reminders of death and of the deceased's passing. Sigmund Freud (1926) was right to note the defensive function of displacement: that which cannot be evaded (e.g., death and the irreversibility of loss) is put out of mind by becoming engrossed with something that *can* be sidestepped. Agoraphobia finds the individual trapped within the home, recoiling from a world in which the deceased no longer lives. Obsessive-compulsive disorder renders the afflicted individual engrossed in concerns about orderliness which can be controlled, as well as dirt and contamination which *can* be scrubbed clean. Panic disorder entails severe responses of physiological stress accompanied by irrational worry that one is dying in the immediate moment, which *can* be allayed with reassurances and avoidance of excitations. Specific phobias, such as fear of dogs or fear of heights, *can* be dealt with through escape. Clients will likely be unwilling to approach personal grief rituals and the dread they stir up if anxiety disorders, with their constricting and debilitating effects, are not treated first.

As discussed in Chapter 2, some bereaved individuals are particularly sensitive to separation anxiety after a loss because they have poor object constancy and cannot maintain healthy continuing bonds with the deceased. This might be due to a long-standing insecure attachment style that makes it challenging to derive comfort from internal mental representations of attachment figures, or the individual may merely exhibit traits of poor object constancy when under the immediate stress of loss. A failure to benefit from experiences of continuing bonds should not be automatic grounds for a psychological diagnosis, but the absence of object constancy can be a symptom of borderline personality disorder, a pervasive malady in which separation anxiety evokes such strong upset that one struggles to cope with the whole of his or her life.

In each anxiety disorder described above, the precipitating stress is, quite plainly, the death of a loved one and subsequent experience of grief. Post-traumatic stress disorder (PTSD) is an exception that requires special consideration. PTSD is *not necessarily a natural reaction to a loss* but commonly stems from specific circumstances that were dangerous, violent, unexpected, frightening, or overwhelming in the moment they occurred. In contrast to the sadness and longing for reunion that is characteristic of unadulterated grief, PTSD yields more of an emotional response of fear marked by intrusive memories that evoke panic as well as persistent anticipation of further dangerous and overwhelming threats that may await in the future, even in lieu of reason to believe that such danger is probable. Additionally, Main and Solomon (1990) augmented Mary Ainsworth's categories of attachment styles by observing a fourth type, *disorganized/unresolved attachment*, where the individual exhibits fearful responses to attachment figures. This type of attachment style has been shown to be highly correlated with a history of relational trauma, including chronic abuse and neglect.

Psychotherapy must be the first line of treatment for bereaved individuals suffering from PTSD. Stroebe's DPM helps us understand why auxiliary interventions such as personalized rituals, as well-intended as they are, may aggravate symptoms of trauma. Personal grief rituals are designed with many factors in mind, one of which is the need to oscillate between loss-oriented stress and restoration-oriented stress. Whichever type of stress is not being coped with sufficiently will be emphasized in the ritual's actions and underlying meaning. But according to the DPM, symptoms of traumatic grief throw a wrench in the wheel of any such plans because of *disturbed oscillations*. At one moment, the traumatized individual is struck by sudden intrusions of overwhelming memories of the traumatic event (loss-oriented stress) followed by, at other moments, dramatic withdrawals from confrontation with the past into states of dissociation. Personal grief rituals that accentuate loss-oriented stress run the risk of plunging the individual into waters that are choppier than they can handle, motivating a panicked retreat into dissociation, thus exacerbating both the intrusive symptoms of trauma and reinforcing problematic avoidance.

Lastly, personal grief rituals often incorporate symbolism into their performance, and these abstractions can confuse certain vulnerable individuals. For instance, those with compromised intellectual functioning may find it hard to understand the meaning behind common ritual behaviors, such as revisiting a meaningful location, releasing ashes into nature, or burning a token that represents something else. Of equal concern are those bereaved individuals who struggle with symptoms of a psychotic disorder, including delusions and hallucinations. Symbolic activity in rituals may prove to be disorienting and disrupt their confidence to distinguish between reality and misperceptions. As an example, many ritual behaviors are designed to afford the bereaved a sense of ongoing connection to the deceased. Imaginary conversations can be held at the grave site, or a plate may be set at the dinner table for a deceased family member. For those struggling with symptoms of schizophrenia and other psychotic disorders, including auditory hallucinations, such rituals threaten to blur the boundaries further between who is actually present and who is not.

The emotionally evocative and symbolic elements of personal grief rituals are generally helpful in facilitating healthy mourning. But for those who are managing additional psychological problems, heightened affect and abstractions carry the potential to further complicate efforts to cope with loss. These potential perils can be mitigated by taking risks into consideration before designing a personal grief ritual and ensuring that they are implemented with caution, care, and rigorous preparation.

Designing the "why" factor of the ritual: Balance, oscillations, temporality, and meaning

A thorough assessment of one's journey through mourning thus far begins to illuminate *why* a particular ritual must be designed for a particular person. The individual's needs and the meaning behind their subjective experience take precedence in its design and performance; the underlying purpose of the ritual (i.e., the "why" factor) takes precedence over the specific behaviors enacted. Thus, a single activity can be used for innumerable purposes for different people. Where one person might design a grief ritual around visiting a grave site to acknowledge the passing of time or to say goodbye, another would use the opportunity to have an illusory conversation with the deceased, and still another individual would reserve that space to conjure up grief and various other emotions. For those who are traversing an unobstructed course of mourning, personal grief rituals will facilitate that which has already come naturally: She expresses and contains emotions as appropriate, confronts absence and relinquishes the past with patience, works towards transitioning into what lies ahead, and establishes a desired degree of continuing bonds. But for those experiencing one form of complicated bereavement or another, *the impediment guides how the ritual is designed.*

Any hindrance usually applies to one of three measures of health: (1) a *balance* of Wordenesque tasks that allow for absence-and-presence (e.g., painful expressions of grief about the deceased's absence and efforts to adapt to life without the deceased are acted upon alongside the comforts of continuing bonds and felt presence), (2) *oscillations* between coping with loss-oriented stress about the loss itself and restoration-oriented stress about what follows, and (3) the *temporality* of how mourning is moving along at a healthy pace, of sustained ambiguity throughout the liminal phase of separating from the past and gradually transitioning into the future.

Worden's task model of mourning is, at its essence, a treatise on the importance of balancing attachment behaviors: *emoting* when distressed (Task II), searching for the lost relationship until accepting absence (Task I), using object constancy to find an internal representation of the deceased (Task IV), and exploring life away from the attachment figure (Task III). This quartet provides four separate answers to the question of *why* one type of ritual would assist the individual more than another. Such a gestalt aids the bereaved when all aspects are balanced and in concert, but lopsided emphasis or neglect on any particular task points towards that which rituals must amplify or abridge.

Activities that actualize the reality of a loss are most notably in order for some. Perhaps the individual has not given sufficient attention towards confronting the stark reality of death and that an important relationship has been lost. Their behaviors, however subtle, suggest they continue to cling to some aspect of the past that needs to be let go. In such instances, personal grief rituals may consist of meaningful acts of separation, opportunities for the bereaved to say goodbye, and confrontations with all that has changed because of the loss.

Van der Hart and Ebbers (1981) distinguished those rites of separation that actualize the reality of loss and permanent absence from those that elicit the painful emotional component of grief. Such rituals enable the bereaved to say goodbye by means of verbalizing grief or by more nonverbal and behavioral expressions of such. Some will require expanded emotional expression, whereas others would benefit from personal grief rituals that *contain and limit* grief.

Anthropologists have come to appreciate that most cultures use rituals to ensure transition to something new for both the deceased and the bereaved. The deceased are to ascend to the next plane of existence while the bereaved, still bound to earth, must carry on being within new roles and identities. Rituals that encourage greater exploration of life after loss provide unique opportunities to actively step into new experiences.

Some bereaved individuals find that continuing bonds are lacking. Whether by dint of a dismissing attachment style that inhibits searching behaviors or a general struggle to access memories of the deceased as desired, these individuals would benefit from rituals that promote a comforting inner bond and a subjective sense that the deceased remains close (Romanoff & Terenzio, 1998). On a similar note, vivid memories of the deceased can be shared among survivors so as to memorialize and affirm the legacy of a valued relationship (Doka, 2012).

But others suffer instead from an excess of presence. They are preoccupied, as it were, with ensuring that the memory of the dead remains accessible, never quite trusting that it can be found again should they step away to engage in life after a loss. The healthy impulse to explore is inhibited and leaves the bereaved stuck and overtly miserable. Personal grief rituals in these cases should aim to loosen ties rather than strengthen that which is already flexed too often.

The DPM and its prescribed oscillations provide yet another framework for conceptualizing why a particular ritual is to be created. A failure to oscillate between loss-oriented and restoration-oriented stresses leaves the bereaved saddled with an excess of one type of stress and a dearth of the other. Personal grief rituals can be designed in a manner that intentionally swings the pendulum towards that which has been neglected. The individual hampered by too much reflection upon the past and unbridled grief about their loss will benefit from activities that emphasize adaptation to the many changes that follow a loss, be it role changes among family and the community, adjustments within one's home, or the pursuit of new endeavors. They are to be drawn out from their sorrowful slumber to gaze upon the dawn that awaits. Conversely, those who have burdened themselves with excessive adaptation can design rituals that put aside time and space to cool one's heels, give pause to reflect upon all that had preceded efforts to find their footing again, and unloose feelings of loss brimming for release.

Temporality, or one's personal relationship to the passing of time, plays a unique role in the subjective experience of loss and grief. The liminal phase of mourning must be sustained long enough to sufficiently step away from the past and gradually ease into the future. Some fail to traverse this ambiguous transition effectively because their pace is too hurried; they arrive at what lies ahead without having committed enough time to truly untether themselves. Others struggle because their lethargic gait has left them bogged down in processes of separation, endlessly wresting themselves from old attachments like so much quicksand. Respectively, personal grief rituals can either be designed to extend the liminal phase of mourning further or constrict it.

Whether the purpose of a personal grief ritual is in service of greater balance, more fluid oscillations, or more even-paced temporality, any act of mourning is invariably grounded in meaning about the individual's subjective experience of loss. The ritual must consist of efforts to give shape and form to the unique significance of an attachment figure's death. Personal grief rituals can certainly be used to confirm and shore up previous systems of meaning-making about mourning (assimilation), but it may be necessary to incorporate novel beliefs, symbols, and behaviors into its performance that help to reconstruct what the loss means to the individual (accommodation). A *constructivist perspective* asserts that loss can create incongruence between previously held systems of meaning-making and the realities of what a recent loss signifies (Neimeyer et al., 2010). The bereaved is then challenged to reconstruct meaning, and it is Neimeyer's charge that a failure to do so contributes mightily to complicated bereavement.

The following questions can help guide the design of personally meaningful grief rituals: How does the loss of a loved one make the bereaved feel, and what needs to be expressed? Can a death afford growth and open up opportunities to experiment with new social roles and identities? Might it be fruitful to search for a symbolic connection to the deceased even after their physical presence is gone? Is there value in sustaining patience within a state of mourning without hurrying to arrive at its desired conclusion?

Let us return once more to the cases of Leroy and Sabrina to consider how a thorough assessment of balance, oscillations, and temporality informs *why* a particular type of grief ritual is to be designed for a particular individual. Leroy demonstrated a pattern of masked grief marked by numerous imbalances, namely, low emotional expression and a deprivation of continuing bonds. He rarely gave voice to feelings of grief about his wife's death (Task II) and quickly relinquished any ongoing attachment to her (Task IV). This constellation of imbalances represents a downregulated attachment system in which he was repressing separation distress and overemphasizing efforts to adapt to life after a loss (Task III). Indeed, Leroy oscillated too strong in the direction of restoration-oriented stress while sidestepping necessary efforts to also cope with loss-oriented stresses. He cloaked the pain of grief behind work, the pursuit of new romantic partners, and a fresh coat of paint. Ironically, these rushed efforts to get past mourning only left him stuck in the very processes he was trying to circumvent; he felt a nagging sense of unease while at home and was disappointed each time a new romantic partner failed to provide an unconscious, ongoing tie to his wife's personality. In his zeal to move on, Leroy propelled himself through the liminal phase of mourning too quickly in a hurried effort to arrive at the next chapter of his life.

As follows, Leroy would benefit from personal grief rituals that inspire a greater balance of emotional expression and continuing bonds, more oscillations away from restoration-oriented stress and towards coping with loss-oriented stress, and a sustained process of separating from the past and steadily transitioning into the future. He could consider making plans to step away from work and approach reminders of the past that draw out feelings about his wife's absence. He could put aside time to feel close to her in spirit while revisiting locations they once frequented or taking part in activities they once enjoyed together. Or Leroy could create a set of recurring rituals during which he slowly relinquishes symbols of the life he and his wife spent together, says goodbye to her, or makes clear his intentions to find a romantic partner that is not a mere replacement of her.

Sabrina presented a different pattern of imbalances which included heightened emotional expression (Task II) and excessive presence (Task IV). Her attachment system was clearly upregulated as she found herself coping with a disproportionate amount of loss-oriented stress. She remained in a perpetual state of emotional protest. Reminiscences preoccupied her mind and distracted her from necessary accommodations to the reality of her husband's absence (Task III). Ruminations over the past contributed to a protracted phase of liminality, stymying the need to transition through time, beyond the moment of her husband's death.

It would behoove Sabrina to design personal grief rituals that limit emotional expression and continuing bonds, oscillate more towards restoration-oriented stresses, and assume a quicker stride through liminality. She could let out emotions within carefully crafted, time-limited parameters. Alongside the ongoing relationship she maintains with her husband, she could also carve out time to pursue new experiences and new relationships. And she could enact rituals during meaningful times of the year to confront the reality of time passing and to demarcate memories of her husband's presence in the past from future moments marked by his absence.

The "who" of the ritual

Upon establishing the essential purpose and meaning of a personal grief ritual, the bereaved will need to be clear about *who* will participate. Many will choose to perform their unique rituals in solitude. It is also perfectly viable to invite a select gathering of others to participate if so desired. A trusted cousin or sibling could be asked to partake in an activity they will also find meaningful. A group of friends can sneak away after the funeral to perform an auxiliary ritual in remembrance of their friend that formal ceremonies would forbid or look down upon. By folding in the company of those whose beliefs or values do not impinge upon the individual's experience of loss, personal grief rituals can maintain a modicum of the social benefits that would otherwise be scrapped if enacted alone.

A professional counselor or psychologist may be one such person who will have the honor of being involved at various stages of a ritual's design and implementation. The client can collaborate with a therapist and bandy about ideas for how to design a personal grief ritual free from concerns about burdening friends or being encroached upon by family or community members who disapprove of unconventional approaches to mourning. Therapy can also provide ample time and space to experiment with how the ritual is to be played out in the most meaningful manner. And insofar as the therapeutic relationship is warm and nurturing, the bereaved individual may even invite the therapist to bear witness and provide social support as the ritual unfolds.

The "what" of the ritual: symbolism and the personal sacred

Grief is often beyond the reach of what language alone can grasp. Even if verbal communication conveys a whisper of what a death means to the bereaved, and even when talking delivers a dose of catharsis, mere words still fall short in capturing the essence of mourning. It is for this reason that every personal grief ritual is enriched by including symbolic objects and actions that embody the visceral depths of one's experience of loss (Sas & Coman, 2016).

Humankind has long turned to symbolism for a more robust expression of loss and grief. Anthropologists such as Turner (1967, 1969) and Geertz (1960) have sought to understand how different cultures infuse meaning into their death rituals by incorporating activities and objects that represent some crucial aspect of the mourning process, what Durkheim (1965) called *sacred symbolism*. The Jewish practice of *keriah*, of rending clothes worn to a funeral, represents the heart-wrenching feeling of a loved one being torn away. Taoists in China embrace the reality of death and loss by burning written announcements; it is believed that the unfurling smoke and ash will reach the land of the dead and act as formal notification of the deceased's departure from the world of the living. And in the Hispanic tradition of *Dia de los Muertos*, food and beverages are shared in a meal with the dead, thus maintaining an abstract ongoing connection with deceased family members.

The body proves to be one of the most potent symbols at the center of many cultures' rituals. Various peoples, including those of Jewish and Hindu culture, implore bereaved family members to bathe and anoint the deceased's body for burial or cremation; when appropriate, the living might also dress the dead in special clothing. These activities typically represent efforts to prepare the dead for transition into the next world. And upon feeling the quickness with which the corpse turns cold and still, the body's changing form drives home a loved one's absence. The Malagasy people of Madagascar continue to interact with the decomposing corpse during *famadihana* rituals for years until the slow process of decay is complete; this corporeal symbol of death's eventual arrival signals that the bereaved are ready to finally cease mourning and reincorporate themselves more fully back into life.

The dead's remains can also provide a powerful symbol that provides an ongoing sense of presence. The ancient Nazca society of Peru threaded rope through the skulls of the deceased, which were then strung along their belts. They also performed mummifications for the purpose of keeping the dead nearby, unlike the ancient Egyptians, whose similar rituals emphasized transmigration of the soul *away* from the living (Lasaponara et al., 2016). Remnants of the body have always been kept proximal and will continue to be held close as the bereaved move forward with their lives, be it a skull hanging from a belt or an urn filled with cremation ashes that presides over the dining room table.

Those in mourning may even be expected to use their own body to signify culturally sanctioned expressions of mourning. Cutting of one's hair acts as an outward acknowledgment of loss. Receiving a tattoo on one's skin provides some with continuing bonds. Some peoples engage in acts of self-injury during funerals to put complex feelings of grief on display. In a particularly shocking representation of separation and emotional pain, the Dani tribe from West Papua New Guinea once performed a finger amputation ritual, now prohibited, in which a surviving spouse was required to cleave off a finger in a public show of sorrow and suffering (Heider, 2017).

But culture sometimes furnishes the individual with symbols that hold no personal value. Or the society in which one is embedded fails to provide access to those symbols that would represent some aspect of their mourning process. As noted previously, American culture has become so gripped with corporeal anxiety and averse to the physical realities of death that its rituals restrict meaningful interactions with the bodies of deceased loved ones. American customs have effectively removed the body from mourning. The individual frustrated with what culture does or does not offer may be better off looking elsewhere for symbols that resonate with what their loss means to them and what their experience of grief feels like.

Durkheim (1965) observed how any object can become socially defined as a sacred symbol as long as it is incorporated into a collective ritual. The individual's experience, however, is all too often treated as undeserving of any reverence and will continue to be relegated to the inferior ranks of the profane. This is precisely why many individuals would benefit from abandoning traditional symbols and striking out to create their own. Whereas the sacred symbolism of collective practices is imbued with agreed-upon meaning for the purpose of binding communities together, the *personal sacred* entails what is profound and meaningful within the individual's unique journey through mourning.

Carl Jung (1964) wrote extensively about how symbols convey crucial information from the depths of the psyche that is otherwise out of reach through language. Whatever emerges within a person's thoughts and dreams is one part collective unconscious, a cache of accumulated images and meaning across culture and throughout time, one part personal and specific to that individual's context and subjective experience. According to Jung, accessing this well of meaning aids the individual in achieving greater psychic wholeness and equilibrium. Fleeting thoughts and images that crop up into conscious awareness act as shorthand substitutes that grasp the complexity of the outer world as it is represented within one's inner world; this is why specific objects and activities resonate with each person in unique ways. And in mourning, the bereaved can use symbolic objects and activities in ritual to give external form to the inner turmoil of loss and make manifest what words alone cannot touch. It would behoove those searching for meaningful representations of grief and mourning to look closely at the images that emerge within their dreams and meandering thoughts.

Generic symbols – clanging of bells, rending of cloth, or veneration of holy scripture – are part and parcel of cultural grief rituals that can create a sense of stale ceremonialism. The bereaved may be better off using personal grief rituals to guide their hand towards objects and symbols within their reach that hold special meaning to them, particularly in regard to *the nature of the relationship they lost*: keepsakes from cherished memories, household items used often by the deceased, wedding rings, gifts and letters from the departed, remnants of their hobbies and pastimes, photographs of the deceased during healthier times, or items of clothing. Intangible symbols can be included as well: specific locations where significant events occurred, a favorite song, or those activities that always brought the bereaved and the now-departed together. Any such object or behavior has the potential to be endowed with a sacred air. Thus, by creating a personal grief ritual, the sacred symbols of the collective are supplanted by those of the *personal sacred*.

Symbols are the concrete elements of a ritual (the "what" that is used in the ritual) that facilitate its designed purpose (the "why" factor). Psychotherapists can certainly play an important role in helping bereaved clients identify the most powerful symbolic actions and objects that address their specific needs (Palazzoli et al., 1978; Van der Hart, 1983), but the professional should insist that it is the client who ultimately selects which items or activities are to be used (Wyrostok, 1995). This ensures that performance of the ritual centers on what is genuinely sacred to the individual and not what the professional envisages as a clever but ultimately generic and insipid symbol.

One of the greatest benefits of ritual lies in their capacity to give form to the abstraction of positive continuing bonds. Rituals can use symbols that invite a healthy compromise between the objective reality of absence and the subjective experience of an ongoing connection, what Winnicott referred to as transitional objects. Whatever item or behavior is chosen, a crucial question must be answered: Does the symbol evoke positive continuing bonds that can be held on to, or does it represent a negative and unhealthy continuing bond that should be relinquished through ritual?

For those bereaved individuals who struggle with insufficient presence, symbols are incorporated into the ritual so as to revive memories and encourage an illusory connection to the deceased. Meaningful actions and objects translate the persistent drive to remain proximal to the attachment figure into something that can be seen, felt, and heard. But for those plagued by excessive presence, who are clinging to concrete objects with unrelenting fear and separation anxiety, symbolism within the ritual must aim to magnify absence and emphasize acts of separation and distance from certain objects. Some symbols will bear a fetish quality that only serve to deny reality, what Volkan (1972) referred to as linking objects. These objects are psychologically defensive in nature, as they are primarily used not to gently mourn a death but, instead, to deny loss and manage separation anxiety by perpetually touching and looking at the item that symbolically represents the deceased. These symbols should not be included in a personal grief ritual as they are likely to only perpetuate complications in the mourning process.

The "where" and "when" of the ritual

One of the more noteworthy functions of the symbolic objects and actions described above is that they flag a ritual as something apart from the mundane. The sight of a holy cross, of mirrors draped in linens, the smell of candles or incense or smudged herbs burning, or the active releasing of ashes into the wind all signal that one has stepped into a ritualistic mindset, a shift of consciousness that distinguishes an extraordinary way of thinking, feeling, and being. Similarly, the specific space and time in which a personal grief ritual is performed pull the bereaved out of the doldrums of day-to-day life and into a sacred context set aside for mourning. Where and when the ritual occurs delimit its boundaries and embed grief and mourning within a spatiotemporal framework with no uncertainty as to why the bereaved is standing in a particular location at a particular time.

Decisions abound regarding *when* the personal grief ritual is to be performed. It is helpful to begin by considering those times of the year that are pregnant with potential meaning: anniversaries, birthdays, holidays, and family traditions. With the cadence of the seasons come familiar sights, sounds, and smells that rekindle memories of the deceased and reawaken feelings of loss associated with a particular moment on the calendar. Upon choosing an important or evocative date, a specific time frame demarcates a clear beginning and end to the ritual. But it need not be limited to one performance. As Rando (1985) advised, rituals can involve a singular event or an ongoing, repetitive act with reiterations at various times throughout the year.

Lastly, the bereaved must decide *where* the ritual will take place. Personal grief rituals can certainly be performed in neutral spaces, as is the case when a psychotherapist offers the therapeutic office as a safe context in which the bereaved can realize their experience of loss and mourning. But the bereaved often have a marked intuition about those specific locations that hold meaning for them, be it a childhood home, an old haunt where the bereaved had spent innumerable hours with the deceased, a place that held meaning for the deceased themselves, or the very sight of their death. Even if an initial trial run of a personal grief ritual is played out within a therapy session, the benefits of such are magnified when immersed in those corners of the world where greater personal significance resides.

Many individuals yearn to mourn outside among the elements of nature, away from the sterile confines of a house or therapy office. Air, earth, water, wind, and fire can all be incorporated by visiting meaningful locations and interacting with tangible symbols among nature. The bereaved regularly feel drawn towards one element or another. Bonfires rage with anger and cathartic release. Rivers, lakes, and ponds may be experienced as cleansing or as facilitating a greater sense of flow and freedom. Throwing ashes into the wind or using symbolism to let go of balloons opens up otherwise bottled-up desires for release, movement, and distance. The bereaved may even wish to act on an urge to touch dirt or burry items beneath the soil.

Why not?: Exploring the individual's resistance to a healthier mourning process

It is a great tragedy that most individuals hesitate to engage in actions that could help them better manage grief and mourning. Just as it is crucial to understand *why* a particular ritual carries the potential to aid the bereaved and counter what thwarts them, it is equally important to understand *why they may not wish to partake in their design and enactment.* Personal grief rituals, though replete with creativity and tailored to the individual's needs, will nonetheless strike some as odd and unconventional. To enter into an unfamiliar sequence of activities challenges the individual's faith in something culture has not repeatedly tested over time. Furthermore, as noted earlier in Chapter 1, mere mention of the word "ritual" may evoke associations to weird, mystical, and irrational behaviors rooted in superstition and primitive beliefs. This is no more apparent than in those expressions of mourning that aim to strengthen a subjective sense of connection to the dead through continuing bonds, which may pique suspicion that one is being lulled into a séance.

Some are averse to even consider participating in rituals for fear of being overwhelmed with a flood of painful emotions. And it is not uncommon for the bereaved to experience moral conflicts and feelings of guilt about using ritual to help them transition into a new life after a loss; they often worry that any improvement or change would amount to a betrayal, a gesture suggesting that the absence of a loved one apparently does not yield much upset. And still, others are more concerned that rituals which encourage forward movement into the future will blur reflections on the past and create a further sense of distance from cherished memories of the dead.

Despite overt hesitations, both the bereaved individual and the professional offering assistance should keep their eyes open and their ears peeled for subtle clues that suggest genuine strivings for a unique approach to mourning. The bereaved may shy away from saying what they desire, but their spontaneous gestures point towards what would be healing. Some will gesticulate as if pushing something away, channeling a need for greater distance and absence. Some will motion as if or pulling something in closer, or they will turn their body towards a vacant spot in the room and begin talking to the deceased, all signaling a wish for greater presence. The bereaved may feel compelled to visit meaningful locations or interact with inanimate objects tied to the past. If not inquired into with genuine curiosity and respect, the bereaved is quick to disregard these impulses as pointless and devoid of meaning – the fanciful wishes of a child.

Raw and inchoate in their fledgling state, the bereaved may be minimally aware of the meaning behind such unprompted behaviors. Those assisting in the design of personal grief rituals can help the individual articulate a more conscious understanding of what their impulses and fleeting thoughts reveal about what they need in order to mourn. By incorporating these spontaneous gestures into a formal ritual with greater intention, the bereaved may come to a better understanding of *why* they manifested in the first place.

Leroy and I eventually created a ritual in which he would once again paint his home in colors akin to his wife's liking. The idea was born out of a moment when he found himself mimicking the slow and deliberate technique his wife used to paint. Leroy squinted his eyes while demonstrating how she used a short handle so that she could get her face close to the wall to inspect her work. I shared a simple observation: Leroy was grinning uncontrollably, like a teenager revealing a furtive crush. That was the first time he divulged his lingering wish to feel closer to her memory, and so the design of his personal grief ritual began.

The work Sabrina and I were doing in therapy took a decisive U-turn when she shared a powerful daydream from the previous day. A small sparrow had managed to fly into the restaurant where she worked and could not find its way out. Sabrina was immediately preoccupied with its whereabouts, consumed by thoughts about how it got inside, whether it was hungry and how the staff might be able to offer the poor bird something to feed on, and how the little sparrow could be let free. She stayed an hour after her shift had ended to continue monitoring the situation. To her surprise, she began crying while relaying her story to me. Sabrina emitted a mixture of embarrassment and confusion in her voice as she recounted a creeping sense of suffocation while watching the bird linger in the rafters. She began imagining that the bird would never leave the restaurant and that, moving forward, she would be distracted by it every time she came back to work another shift. Sabrina put up her hands and gestured as if trying to bat away something close to her face. She said, "I just wanted to go home and talk to my friends. I didn't want to be stuck there anymore. And that's when my husband popped into my head." Sabrina still wanted to hold on to memories of the love of her life and the father of her children, but at that moment, she was able to recognize an equal yearning to move on, to no longer be caged within memories of the past. It was at that precise moment when we first talked about how she wanted to begin getting rid of his clothes.

To create and embody a personal grief ritual is nothing short of a courageous act. Trepidation and uncertainty accompany the bereaved as they journey down a path no one else has treaded upon. And cultural grief rituals remain ever-present, beckoning the individual to fall back into the comforting lap of what is tried and true. Furthermore, acting out a one-man show of grief can be lonely; as anthropologists and psychologists over the past century have observed, feelings of connectedness and solidarity pull the majority back to participate in collective grief rituals once again (Durkheim, 1965; Imber-Black, 1991; Radcliffe-Brown, 1964). But for many, the potential costs of joining the masses – exhibition of disingenuous emotions, a prolonged phase of liminality that thwarts forward movement, excessive or insufficient opportunities for continuing bonds – far outweigh the benefits of familiarity and social cohesion. And so the individual may choose to march forward bravely into the unknown, to abandon the path carved out by culture and blaze their own trail en route to a more meaningful experience of mourning. As Rudyard Kipling once said in an interview with Arthur Gordon (1983):

> The individual has always had to struggle to keep from being overwhelmed by the tribe. If you try it, you will be lonely often, and sometimes frightened. But no price is too high to pay for the privilege of owning yourself. (p. 7)

References

Alexiou, M. (1974). *The ritual lament in Greek tradition.* Cambridge University Press.

Al-Krenawi, A. (1999). An overview of rituals in Western therapies and intervention. *International Journal for the Advancement of Counselling, 21*(1), 3–17.

Birx, H. J. (2006). *Encyclopedia of anthropology.* SAGE Publications.

Bolton, C., & Camp, D. J. (1987). Funeral rituals and the facilitation of grief work. *OMEGA – Journal of Death and Dying, 17*(4), 343–352.

Budiman, M. (2013). *Contemporary funeral rituals of Sa'dan Toraja: From Aluk Todolo to "new" religions.* Karolinum Press.

Castle, J., & Phillips, W. L. (2003). Grief rituals: Aspects that facilitate adjustment to bereavement. *Journal of Loss & Trauma, 8*(1), 41–71.

Coleman, R. A., & Neimeyer, R. A. (2010). Measuring meaning: Searching for and making sense of spousal loss in later life. *Death Studies, 34,* 804–834.

Doka, K. J. (2012). Therapeutic ritual. In R. Neimeyer (Ed.), *Techniques of grief therapy: Creative practices for counseling the bereaved* (pp. 341–343). Routledge.

Durkheim, E. (1965). *The elementary forms of the religious life* (Joseph Ward Swain, Trans. & Ed.). Free Press.

Fiese, B., Tomcho, T., Douglas, M., Josephs, K., Poltrock, S., & Baker, T. (2002). A review of 50 years of research on naturally occurring family routines and rituals. *Journal of Family Psychology, 16*(4), 381–390.

Freud, S. (1926). Inhibitions, symptoms, and anxiety. *Standard Edition, 20,* 75–174. Hogarth Press.

Fulton, R. (1988). Death and the funeral in contemporary society. In H. Wass (Ed.), *Dying: Facing the facts* (pp. 236–255). Hemisphere Publishing Corp.
Geertz, C. (1960). *The religion of Java*. Free Press.
Gordon, A. (1983). Six hours with Rudyard Kipling. In H. Orel (Ed.), *Kipling: Interviews and recollections* (Vol. 2, pp. 5–8). Palgrave Macmillan.
Grimes, R. L. (2004). Consuming ritual: A&E's sacred rites and rituals. In C. C. Otnes & T. M. Lowrey (Eds.), *Contemporary consumption rituals: A research anthology* (1st ed., pp. 21–36). Lawrence Erlbaum Associates.
Heider, K. G. (2017). *The Dugum Dani: A Papuan culture in the highlands of West New Guinea*. Taylor & Francis.
Huggins, C. L., & Hinkson, G. M. (2019). Contemporary burial practices in three Caribbean islands among Christians of African descent. *OMEGA – Journal of Death and Dying, 80*(2), 266–279.
Imber-Black, E. (1991). Rituals and the healing process. In F. Walsh & M. McGoldrick (Eds.), *Living beyond loss: Death in the family* (pp. 207–223). WW Norton & Comp.
Johnston, S. (1999). *Restless dead: Encounters between the living and the dead in ancient Greece*. University of California Press.
Jung, C. (1964). *Man and his symbols*. Doubleday.
Lasaponara, R., Masini, N., & Orefici, G. (2016). *The ancient Nasca world: New insights from science and archaeology*. Springer Publishing Company.
Laungani, P. (1997). Death in a Hindu family. In P. Laungani & W. Young (Eds.), *Death and bereavement across cultures* (pp. 52–72). Routledge.
Lofland, L. (1985). The social shaping of emotion. *Symbolic Interaction, 8*(2), 171–190.
Main, M., & Solomon, J. (1990). Procedures for identifying infants as disorganized/disoriented during the Ainsworth Strange Situation. In M. T. Greenberg, D. Cicchetti, & E. M. Cummings (Eds.), *Attachment in the preschool years: Theory, research, and intervention* (p. 121–160). University of Chicago Press.
Metcalf, P., & Huntington, R. (1991). *Celebrations of death: The anthropology of mortuary ritual*. Cambridge University Press.
Neimeyer, R. A., Burke, L. A., Mackay, M. M., & van Dyke Stringer, J. G. (2010). Grief therapy and the reconstruction of meaning: From principles to practice. *Journal of Contemporary Psychotherapy, 40*(2), 73–83.
Norton, M. I., & Gino, F. (2014). Rituals alleviate grieving for loved ones, lovers, and lotteries. *Journal of Experimental Psychology, 143*(1), 266–272.
Palazzoli, M. S., Boscolo, L., Cecchin, G., & Prata, G. (1978). *Paradox and counterparadox: A new model in the therapy of the family in schizophrenic transaction*. Jason Aronson, Inc.
Platvoet, J. G. (1995). Ritual in plural and pluralist societies: Instruments for analysis. In J. G. Platvoet & K. Toorn (Eds.), *Pluralism and identity: Studies in ritual behaviour* (pp. 25–51). E. J. Brill.
Rabkin, R. (1977). *Strategic psychotherapy*. Basic Books.
Radcliffe-Brown, A. (1964). *The Andaman islanders*. Free Press.
Rando, T. A. (1985). Creating therapeutic rituals in the psychotherapy of the bereaved. *Psychotherapy, 22*, 236–240.
Reeves, N. C. (2011). Death acceptance through ritual. *Death Studies, 35*(5), 408–419.
Romanoff, B. D., & Terenzio, M. (1998). Rituals and the grieving process. *Death Studies, 22*(8), 697–711.
Sas, C., & Coman, A. (2016). Designing personal grief rituals: An analysis of symbolic objects and actions. *Death Studies, 40*(9), 558–569.

Schachter, S. R., & Finneran, K. M. (2013). Expansion of new rituals for the dying and bereaved. In C. Staudt & J. Ellens (Eds.), *Our changing journey to the end: Reshaping death, dying, and grief in America* (pp. 165–192). ABS-CLIO, LLC.

Schenck, L. K., Eberle, K. M., & Rings, J. A. (2016). Insecure attachment styles and complicated grief severity: Applying what we know to inform future directions. *OMEGA – Journal of Death and Dying, 73*(3), 231–249.

Stroebe, M., & Schut, H. (1999). The dual process model of coping with bereavement: Rationale and description. *Death Studies, 23*, 197–224.

Stroebe, M., & Schut, H. (2016). Overload: A missing link in the dual process model? *OMEGA – Journal of Death and Dying, 74*(1), 96–109.

Swarts, E. D. (2001). *Kaimyo (Japanese Buddhist posthumous names) as indicators of social status* (Publication No. 3022582) [Doctoral dissertation, The Ohio State University]. ProQuest Dissertations Publishing.

Turner, V. (1967). *The forest of symbols*. Cornell University Press.

Turner, V. (1969). *The ritual process*. Aldine.

Van der Hart, O. (1983). *Rituals in psychotherapy: Transition and continuity*. Irvington.

Van der Hart, O., & Ebbers, J. (1981). Rites of separation in strategic psychotherapy. *Psychotherapy: Theory, Research & Practice, 18*(2), 188–194.

van Gennep, A. (1960). *The rites of passage*. University of Chicago Press.

Volkan, V. D. (1972). The linking objects of pathological mourners. *Archives of General Psychiatry, 27*(2), 215–221.

Walter, T. (1996). Facing death without tradition. In P. C. Jupp & G. Howarth (Eds.), *Contemporary issues in the sociology of death, dying, and disposal* (pp. 193–204). Palgrave Macmillan.

Wilson, G. (1939). Nyakyusa conventions of burial. *Bantu Studies, 13*, 1–31.

Wojtkowiak, J., Lind, J., & Smid, G. E. (2021). Ritual in therapy for prolonged grief: A scoping review of ritual elements in evidence-informed grief interventions. *Frontiers in Psychiatry, 11*, 623835. VOLUME=11. https://doi.org/10.3389/fpsyt.2020.623835

Worden, J. W. (2008). *Grief counseling and grief therapy: A handbook for the mental health practitioner* (4th ed.). Springer Publishing Company.

Wouters, C. (2002). The quest for new rituals in dying and mourning: Changes in the we-I balance. *Body & Society, 8*(1), 1–27.

Wyrostok, N. (1995). The ritual as a psychotherapeutic intervention. *Psychotherapy: Theory, Research, Practice, Training, 32*(3), 397–404.

Chapter 4

Confirming absence

Rituals that facilitate acceptance of loss

Rick squints his eyes and stares at the patterned rug in my office as he recalls, with an air of confusion, a dream he had the previous night. He and his friend are eating lunch together at one of their favorite haunts on a typical Wednesday in downtown Milwaukee; this was the tradition they held for nearly fifteen years. Rick orders a sandwich. His friend, as she always did, orders a salad. The banality of what he reports leads me to clarify whether he is telling me about the dream or a memory, to which he responds, "Both, I suppose." I ask him to describe how he experienced the dream. Was it frightening? Sad? Did a sense of calm rush over him? Rick shrugs his shoulders and raises his hands in befuddlement, saying, "It's just what we used to do, exactly the same as how things were before she . . ." Rick truncates his answer and abruptly returns his gaze to the rug.

Carina, who I had been seeing in therapy for a year following the death of her husband, begins the session as she often does, by saying, "I keep having the same goofy dream." I offer, "The one where you wake up next to Leonard and he is still alive?" Carina's eyes fill with tears. Her emotional response to my use of the words "still alive" suggests more than sadness. Her jaw tightens. She purses her lips. Carina is angry and frustrated with me.

Jocelyn, in her characteristically dry and matter-of-fact tone, reports a recent dream during which she walks into the garage of her father's house to find him standing at the workbench they built together many years ago. They proceed to do handiwork around the house side by side, just as they had always done. Nothing unusual happens. Jocelyn's dreams are synonymous with memories exactly as they occurred prior to the day she received a phone call informing her that her father had died from cardiac arrest while taking a walk in the neighborhood. Her affect is notably flat; she is nonchalant as she shares this with me, as if making small talk about the weather.

Denial: Defense and adaptation

In mourning, all roads lead back to the imperative task of accepting reality. Shock and disconnect from the poignancy of grief are commonplace

DOI: 10.4324/9781351204873-4

immediately after a loss. Denial can even be respected as an adaptive response early on, a buffer against overwhelming and harsh upsets. But absolute repudiation of death usually proves to be short-lived. The shield erodes steadily to the persistent assault of reality. And yet the stark truth of the matter does not set in as quickly or as decisively as one would imagine. Even when the disquieting realization of absence begins to dawn, its light shines only partially. The battered shield remains in hand, giving the bereaved a thin sliver of shadow behind which they continue to hide.

Sigmund Freud (1926) spoke of how the mind is essentially split in two in its effort to accept the reality of a death, simultaneously holding a representation of the deceased being absent, and of the deceased remaining present. Myriad behaviors throughout mourning demonstrate this ambivalence. For instance, each of the individuals referenced above would plainly admit that their loved ones have passed; they did, after all, willingly bring themselves in for therapy because of loss and grief. And at the same time, they are continually working to accommodate reality into their daily perceptions. Rick hesitates to articulate that his friend "died." Carina is frustrated by anything or anyone that reminds her of her husband's absence. Jocelyn's affect suggests that her grief is still so painful as to motivate utter detachment from emotion. The manifest content of each of their dreams is emblematic of one of the more central tensions experienced early in mourning: the unconscious wish to deny the passing of time, preserve the past, and once more find their loved ones as they had always been. One of my mentors from graduate school, Dr. Johanna Tabin, quipped in an unpublished interview at the end of her life about the prompt response of protest against loss that is hard-wired in us all, as well as the inevitable resignation that follows:

> *Well, you can't have restitution . . . if there is a spot on my white dress when I'm two years old, I will scream and scream and scream, that dress is gone, lost. Oh, I can myself get rid of it, get a little cloth and wipe it off. But it will never again be that white dress.*

Why does denial of loss persist with such tenacity? How could it be that perceptions and cognitions remain recalcitrant in the face of overwhelming evidence that loved ones are no longer present? The answer, quite simply, is that it is noxious to confront the absolute finality of death. Acceptance paves the way for distressing grief and anxiety. Plus, each death stokes awareness of our own personal mortality and the transience of everyone and everything we encounter. Being reminded that our bodies will steadily decline towards decay is demoralizing. If we do look at death, it is, as Irvin Yalom has suggested, akin to staring at the sun: We can only stare so long before it burns us. And so it is oddly beneficial to avert our gaze, to be at least partially blind to death, lest our efforts to concentrate on work or enjoy time with friends and family are spoiled by morbid thoughts and a sense of ultimate futility.

At times, denial only obscures select facts or circumstances about the loss that are hard to look upon. For example, the bereaved may be fully capable of accepting that a loved one has died but still struggles to speak of *how* they passed. Certain causes of death are more difficult to think about than others, such as suicides, stillbirths, violent homicide, drug overdoses, or death as the result of AIDS-related disorders. Or it may be the meaning of a particular loss that we turn away from. The bereaved might avoid conscious contemplation of there being no further chances to develop the kind of relationship with a parent they had always hoped for, or how the loss of a spouse will impact the children as they grow up, or that the family lineage has come to an end.

American culture grants the bereaved permission to avert their gaze, but many will still feel another instinct tugging at them, a healthy counterbalance that tempts one to look death square in the eyes. On November 22, 1963, just two quick hours after her husband had been assassinated, Jackie Kennedy appeared on television with Lyndon Johnson as he was sworn into office. She insisted upon wearing the same bloodstained pink suit she had on when her husband was shot and killed at her side. Jackie made no effort to clean up before appearing on air. In that moment, she intuited that the country, already in a state of shock, needed to see the reality of what happened. And as America found themselves staring at their televisions in disbelief, participating in an improvised ritual confirming the sudden absence of their president, not one person could look away from the truth.

Persistent denial and complicated bereavement

Occasional rifts between reality and repudiation of death are not necessarily problematic. There will be moments, however brief, when the bereaved seem to forget about loss and behave as if their loved ones are still alive. They may even struggle to find the words that align with the finality of their loss, lapsing instead into present tense when conversing about the dead. The ever-present use of cellular phones in modern times has given rise to a new symptom of fleeting denial: Those reeling from a recent death often catch themselves picking up their phones and going through the motions to call the person they have lost, realizing the absurdity of their behavior only after noticing their thumb hovering over the deceased's name. Like ocean waves that steadily erode the shore, those in mourning are surprised to encounter one reminder after the other that the relationship that grounded them for so long has been swept out to sea.

But denial can persist beyond the pale and yield costly complications. Grief left unaddressed nonetheless finds expression through some path of least resistance and rears its head in physical pains and somatoform ailments, such as headaches, ulcers, and eliminative problems. Reminders of loss within the home and in the community are avoided for fear of piquing strong emotions. And by doing so, the bereaved deprive themselves of opportunities to adapt and move forward. Visiting a house or workplace where the deceased regularly frequented, taking part in activities reminiscent of how the bereaved used to spend time with the departed, or using possessions that once belonged to them – any of these may come to represent an anxious cue to confront a reality from which the bereaved would rather hide away.

Such refusal to accommodate reality is problematic for entire bereft families. Crucial roles once performed by the deceased are left vacant. They may have provided spiritual guidance, managed financial concerns, served as a beacon of calm and wisdom during tough times, or helped organize large family gatherings. If the bereaved decline to assume these empty positions, because doing so would trigger harsh reminders of absence, the void is swept under the rug and the next family gathering goes unplanned.

It is uniquely challenging for someone from a younger generation to shoulder the responsibilities of an older figure whose strength, wisdom, and confidence once acted as a bulwark against life's hardships. Ernest Becker (1973) spoke of how humans strive to stand out as special and be heroic in defiance of death but find that the task looms too large. Sobering reminders of one's smallness accumulate, and in a last-ditch effort to stand up to mortality, a more powerful individual is cast as a symbol of invulnerability, someone with whom one can merge and feel strong by proxy. But when death inevitably takes them away, how unsettling it is to no longer be able to lean upon larger-than-life figures to protect us from all that is uncertain in life. What a shock to see those who once protected and guided us through life now lying enfeebled in a hospital bed or defeated in a casket. And what is more, to assume those vacant roles demands that the bereaved come to terms with the fact that even one's heroes were not able to evade death's wrathful sickle, just as they will suffer the same fate. All too often, survivors prefer instead to perpetuate a stance of helplessness and instinctively cower in quiet hopes of their omnipotent attachment figures returning to provide protection once more.

Additionally, it is not uncommon to find the bereaved attempting to soothe the pains of loss by supplanting the deceased with a new spouse or a new friend or a new father figure that affords the illusion of nothing having changed. In the controversial fictional novel *Lolita*, for instance, the protagonist Humbert Humbert copes with the devastating death of his first childhood love by perpetually searching for a youthful replacement, an increasingly inappropriate love object as he becomes older: "The ache remained with me, and that little girl with her seaside limbs and ardent tongue haunted me ever since – until at last, twenty-four years later, I broke her spell by incarnating her in another" (Nabokov, 1997, p. 15).

Social withdrawal is one of the most problematic outgrowths of denial and avoidance. Many people struggle to mourn primarily because they keep their distance from the very relationships that could provide much-needed support. Indeed, research shows that the bereaved fare better if they perceive their relationships to be providing adequate support (Stroebe & Schut, 1999), if they are in regular contact with people who knew the deceased and are mourning the same loss (Worden, 2008), and if they participate in more and varied social roles (Hershberger & Walsh, 1990). But contact with others is a double-edged sword that inevitably invites confrontations with the reality of loss. Questions of "How are you doing?" convey that there is much to be upset about. Even the nonverbal shows of compassion in the faces of friends and family mirror the bereaved individual's pain. And stories about the deceased, those reminders of all that has been lost, will be ripe for the telling. Merely being in the presence of others is enough to highlight who is no longer there.

Per Emile Durkheim and the many cultural anthropologists who followed, one of the most crucial functions of cultural grief rituals is that they bring people together to provide emotional support in times of loss and mourning and acknowledge what the psyche naturally wishes to banish out of conscious awareness: the unpleasant reality of a loved one's absence. Take, for example, the Japanese Obon festival, also known as the Bon Odori. An irreducibly collective society, Japan has rituals that emphasize an inherent unity among those in mourning rather than a sole focus on a singular family's experiences. Dating back 1,500 years, the Obon festival occurs during the fall equinox and invites families to visit the graves of family members and honor their memory together (Saito, 2014).

The vast majority of mourning rituals throughout the world involve social interaction as their cornerstone: The bereaved gather to acknowledge their mutual losses. Most individuals will take part in such customs at some point throughout life, whether attending an Irish wake, a funeral, or the Jewish custom of sitting shiva. And yet as previously discussed, some mourners do not have access to larger social supports and cultural practices. Culture can also fail to confront a specific aspect of the personal meaning behind an individual's loss that they need to face. In place of the collective, personal grief rituals can be designed to help the individual confirm the reality of loss and absence on their own.

The attachment perspective: Confronting absence by looking back or by looking ahead

In the pages that follow, we will take a look at various individuals who designed personal grief rituals to confront some facet of loss they had failed to square up to. Attachment theory tells us that those with a secure attachment style will not likely be in great need of such activities, as they are less likely to evade unpleasant thoughts and feelings in the first place. Nonetheless, most people stand to gain from deeper contemplations of loss and absence. Even those with a secure attachment style can capitulate to the stress of grief and turn away from the harsh reality of coping with death. And those who are experiencing an uncomplicated course may still benefit from building meaningful activities into their journey through mourning that acknowledge all that has passed.

No one is altogether ill-suited for personal grief rituals that confirm absence. But each individual should consider the distinct types of stress they need to confront more of and which they have already come to grips with, perhaps in excess. Research on the DPM suggests that loss-oriented and restoration-oriented stress pertain to distinctly different challenges in accommodating reality. Those with a dismissing attachment style, as well as those exhibiting dismissing tendencies while in mourning, tend to neglect loss-oriented confrontations with reality and overemphasize restoration-oriented stress. That is, the stress of what lies ahead is given undue privilege while the past is paid no mind. Thus, they would benefit from rituals that have them face more of the reality of having lost an important relationship who once walked alongside them (e.g., storytelling, looking through photos, revisiting old haunts and reflecting upon the past); they would actually be poorly served by any activity that has them acknowledge even more stress regarding all they need to adapt to. Conversely, those with a preoccupied attachment style, as well as those presenting with preoccupied tendencies, need personal grief rituals that plant their feet in the present moment and help them confront the stress of adapting to all that has changed and been left vacant in the wake of loss (e.g., write/talk to the deceased from the present, interact with the elements of nature to symbolically let go, engage in searching behaviors with the conscious intention of not finding the deceased). The preoccupied individual needs to ensure that they do not saturate themselves further in reflections on the past that are already crowding their mind.

Storytelling: Rekindling memories of the dead to observe the passing of time

If we are to observe the haunting reality of loss and embrace absence, we must first stare down the specter of time. There must be definitive acknowledgment of the fact that those who were once present now reside in memories of the past. It is for this reason that mourning often begins with a formal declaration of death. Obituaries printed in the newspaper have long served this need to inform a community of who has recently passed. And in recent years, the bereaved have turned to social media to share news of a recent loss with a wider audience. It is customary in Chinese culture to place white banners or blue lanterns outside the house to announce a death to the community. Written messages are also burned to notify the gods of the underworld that the deceased's spirit is en route to its final destination (Kiong, 1993).

Beyond these immediate proclamations, the bereaved continue to contemplate the passing of time by dredging up memories. Rituals may center on reminiscences, the observation of important anniversaries, and storytelling so as to ensure that the dead are not forgotten. It might seem as if these meditations on the past only lead the bereaved too far afield into the past, but there is great value in referencing the past *for the sake of confirming that the deceased was once here and that they are no longer present.*

Consider the ubiquitous practice of delivering a eulogy at a funeral service. The ancient Greek scholar and poet Callimachus first crafted a short form of emotive poetry called an elegy, derived from the Greek *eulogia* and translated as "praise." English poets in the Romantic Era of the 1800s built upon this practice with an increasingly mournful tone, and over time, the elegy became known as a eulogy, less of a lyrical poem and more of the spoken act of remembrance and expression of sorrow that many are familiar with today.

Storytelling is the essence of a eulogy. As practiced today, eulogies serve to preserve memories and honor the life left behind. Memorable sayings, references to the deceased's favorite foods and pastimes, outstanding personality traits, funny anecdotes, and major achievements are all regularly shared. A life is conveyed through story and contextualized in the past. In a similar use of ritual described in Chapter 1, the Ojibwe community hold a yearly feast to remember the dead and remind the Ojibwe people that "Death is accepted as a Rite of Passage into the next phase of the soul's journey" (Walker-Gillet, 2011, p. 99).

Personal grief rituals can build off these traditions and use storytelling to rekindle memories in a more private and uninhibited setting, free from the censures of delivering a polite eulogy that does not offend or the stuffy confines of an obituary printed within a small corner of page 37 in the newspaper. Whether through writing or spoken word, the individual can articulate *their own personal memories of the deceased.* This private and personal approach is especially helpful when the public experience of hearing a eulogy fails to address what was important to the bereaved about their particular relationship with the dead.

Whenever I am working with a patient who is crafting a personal grief ritual that features storytelling, I encourage them to make plans to read what they wrote out loud, perhaps in a meaningful location (the "where" of the ritual). Many additional decisions are to be made regarding whom it will be read to, whether by themselves at the deceased's grave site, with a select group of family members at someone's home, or in a psychotherapy session with a therapist. The bereaved may even choose to access social media to make a meaningful statement on the internet about who they lost and the life their loved one lived. It is the individual's choice whether to take this type of ritual public or keep it private; either way, reading a narrative out loud creates a more visceral experience that drives home the reality of a lost relationship.

It is also helpful to include symbols in rituals that evoke fond remembrances and acknowledge the passing of time. Entire nations and small towns alike pay tribute to their fallen leaders or beloved sports heroes with a statue in a park or a display in a museum adorned with inanimate objects – a pen, a baseball bat, a piece of clothing that was worn – reminiscent of a meaningful day in history, all of which capture moments in time that may have otherwise receded into a forgotten past. Even humanity's proclivity for war has given birth to a few noteworthy rituals which, when deployed, give the bereaved a way to make meaning out of loss through remembrance. During the Napoleonic Wars in the early nineteenth century, France's national flag was first draped over coffins of dead soldiers to represent their devotion to country while alive. United States Memorial Day became a federal holiday in 1971, encouraging Americans to carve out time to reflect upon all those who have sacrificed their lives for the sake of country.

Symbols reminiscent of the deceased's life provide an ongoing reminder of what came and went, and the individual in mourning can incorporate any item of their choosing into a more private homage. Pictures of fond memories can be used as decorations throughout the house. The deceased's possessions can be displayed in meaningful places, be it a fishing pole hung above a fireplace in the family cabin where fishing trips once took place or a favorite cooking utensil affixed to a wall in the kitchen. The bereaved can put aside time to look at old pictures, watch family videos, or listen to audio recordings. A man who I will discuss later, Sai, created a personal grief ritual in which he would watch old slide show reels of his father's life every year on his father's birthday, thus giving himself an opportunity to pause and reflect upon a relationship he dearly misses.

In Ghana, particularly among the Ga people residing in Accra, the dead may be buried in *abebu adekai*, or *fantasy coffins*. These are unique and custom-made coffins which act as visual representation of some meaningful aspect of the deceased's life, be it their work, their role in the community, or a beloved hobby (Bonetti, 2019). Examples include a coffin resembling a Mercedes-Benz for a businessman who collected cars, one shaped like a rifle for a hunting enthusiast, and a coffin crafted to look like the Bible for a devout churchgoer. Such artistic and visual reminders of the person's life present the bereaved with an opportunity for remembrance that highlights the personality once exhibited by whoever occupies the very coffin in view.

Any failure to fix memories of the dead squarely in the past leaves the bereaved disoriented as to where they stand. They may feel anchored to nostalgia, as if no time has passed, or they may sense that the clock has wound its hands at a furious pace, creating a terrifying chasm between now and a place in time in which the deceased was still alive. Personal grief rituals can be designed in a manner that is firmly grounded in the current moment while also using storytelling and meaningful symbols to look back.

Jason, a man in his late forties, came in for grief therapy many years after his father died following a prolonged battle with Alzheimer's disease. Jason was of perfectly sound mind but was perturbed to find that memories of the relationship he had with his father were blurry at best. He could not confidently say how long it had been since his father had died. Furthermore, when Jason reflected upon the years that preceded his father's illness, he struggled to recall the many positive times they had shared. He seemed to have no recollection of the activities they did together during his childhood or what they discussed as adults. Jason often uttered, "It sounds crazy, but I still can't believe the old man is actually gone, and I don't know what feels different now." He knew his father was absent, no longer a part of his day-to-day life, but in regard to the relationship they once had, Jason remained uncertain about exactly *what* he had lost.

The decisive moment came when, upon rummaging through a mess of his father's belongings, Jason stumbled upon the very tackle box his father used when they would go fishing together during his childhood. He was immediately revisited by a stream of vivid recollections: waking up early in the morning to the smell of his father brewing coffee, the quiet that hung in the air and the subtle sounds of the water as they sat patiently waiting for a bite to tug on the line, and the long explanations his father provided about which lures to use. Jason began to share these anecdotes in therapy. Still, he felt restless. He wanted to do something to revive his memories further. I suggested that he embody his recollections through a relevant action of sorts, say, fishing or the tackle box that summoned these memories in the first place. Jason responded, "My son has always wanted me to teach him how to fish, just like my dad taught me!" We then began making plans for him to take his son out on the water, teach him how to use the various lures in the tackle box, and regale him with stories of his grandfather and the adventures they enjoyed early in the morning. Jason always had an infectious smile, and I can still picture the grin on his face when he told me he had decided to hand down his father's tackle box to his son.

Death anniversaries: When to reignite memories

Cultural rites and rituals typically occur in the days immediately after death, prompting a swift confrontation with reality and acceptance of loss. But ritual can also be used to observe anniversaries and other significant dates throughout the year well after the immediate wounds of grief have begun to heal. The bereaved, as well as those in their community, often rationalize that mourning should have subsided in full as time goes by and that any further focus on losses during anniversaries, birthdays, or holidays is superfluous. Regardless, the calendar demands recognition. Anniversaries coax out pronounced feelings of emptiness, absence, and pining for reunion that may have laid dormant through less-significant seasons. This phenomenon speaks volumes to the depths of grief that lie in wait within the unconscious realm of the mind, as well as the benefits of voluntarily confronting the thoughts and feelings that arise during meaningful times of the year.

The Catholic celebration of All Saints Day, the Mexican holiday of Dia de los Muertos, and the Japanese ritual of Bon Odori are all examples of how culture reserves time for a community to collectively honor their dead and return once more to a state of remembrance. Many cultures use rituals on or near the specific anniversary of a death, oft referred to as a *death anniversary*, to pause and confront the reality of exactly *when* a significant other died. Roman Catholics celebrate memories of the deceased in Mass near the death anniversary. Chinese traditions of ancestor worship use anniversary dates to pay homage to the dead with prayer and elaborate banquets. In countries where Hinduism is practiced, including Nepal and India, intricate *sraddha* rituals are performed on the death anniversary to express gratitude for all that the deceased provided while they were alive (Cush et al., 2008).

In Judaism, it is tradition to light a *yahrzeit* candle in memory of the deceased on the anniversary of their passing. It is also customary to recite the mourner's Kaddish, a prayer for the dead in celebration of life given by the almighty, during the first year after burial services and at varying intervals of time, depending upon familial practices, sometimes weekly during Sabbath service, and sometimes daily (Levine, 1997). Reciting Kaddish and lighting yahrzeit candles can occur on subsequent anniversaries too. Although each of these rituals has numerous and complex functions, their enactment acts as a meditation on the passing of time and a reminder of who is gone.

The bereaved individual can look to these traditions for inspiration and brainstorm ideas for how to create their own personal grief ritual during meaningful times of the year (the "when" of the ritual). Most importantly, they can be designed around memories and dates most relevant to their personal relationship with the deceased. Candles or incense can be burned to reflect upon annual traditions – attending a sporting event, engaging in outdoor hobbies, or time spent going on vacations – once enjoyed together. The individual can demarcate a moment during the death anniversary to read a prayer or a passage from a favorite book that their loved one also appreciated. Seasonal foods that the deceased and bereaved both liked can be consumed to give pause and commemorate the memory of a loved one's hunger for life.

A brief cautionary note is in order if developing a personal grief ritual based on storytelling or significant dates. Upon digging up the past, the bereaved may end up reviving memories filled with upsetting or morbid details of a loss: observing the visual progression of illness, the shock of receiving news of a sudden loss, or having been present during the precise moment of death. Resurrecting these types of memories sometimes reveals a pattern of thoughts, feelings, and behaviors indicative of post-traumatic stress disorder (PTSD), as discussed in the previous chapter. Those individuals managing such a sequala of symptoms will struggle to root their recall of the past firmly in the present; traumatic memories are all too often experienced *as if they were reoccurring.* While it is true that persistent avoidance of anxiety-producing thoughts, as well as specific locations that trigger intense feelings associated with a loss, does leave the bereaved in a precarious position, personal grief rituals that revisit the past should not be casually thrust upon those beset with PTSD without first establishing intensive psychological treatment.

Writing and talking to the deceased . . . from the present

Writing or talking *about* the deceased helps reclaim memories that can be both moving to recall and bittersweet to acknowledge. Many grief rituals center on such reminiscences and drive home the reality that a once-present relationship is now spoken of in past tense. A slight variation on this approach involves writing or talking *to* the deceased while firmly rooted in the here and now. Whatever topic one chooses to discuss when enacting this type of personal grief ritual, it should be in reference to the weeks, months, and years beyond the deceased's final days, and it should inform the dead about the present moment which they are no longer able to experience. The bereaved may write in a journal as if writing to the dead, hold imaginary conversations with the deceased, or visit a grave site to be the harbinger of updates on the family.

Sai was a man in his late forties whose parents both died suddenly in a tragic car accident when he was twenty-seven years old. Writing had been one of his favorite pastimes ever since childhood. Sai wrote beautiful public obituaries for his parents shortly after their deaths. He also wrote and read part of their eulogy at the joint funeral held for them both. I had already been providing him therapy for two years when he revealed that he always quietly regretted not saying goodbye to his mother and father. I asked him to clarify what he meant. Sai informed me that both of his parents held on to life for a few days after the accident before succumbing to their devastating injuries. He had visited them in the hospital, but out of hope for their recovery, he did not take the opportunity to bid them farewell. We discussed what he would have liked to tell them, and as he held his head in his hands and wept, he said, "I wanted them to know that I would be OK. That they didn't have to worry about me anymore."

A few weeks after that appointment, Sai informed me that he and his wife and their two children were planning a trip to spend time with family who lived in the town where his parents were buried. I invited him to consider using the opportunity to visit their graves and let them know how he was doing. Ever the writer, Sai decided to pen an update for his parents about his life that he could read at their grave sites before bidding them farewell, as he had always wished he would have done. He asked me if he could read what he had written aloud in my office before sharing it with his parents. Sai recited it to me in the next session, and when he finished, I was floored to hear him say, "I still feel like I have never really said goodbye to them, like they are still waiting for me." Before he left, we talked about exactly how he wanted to structure his time visiting their resting places. Sai stated that, before reading to them in private, he would find great meaning in first introducing his wife and children. "To let them know they would have had a daughter-in-law, and grandchildren, and that we are all doing OK."

There is a crucial distinction between this type of personal grief ritual, which clearly acknowledges the deceased's absence, and those that invoke continuing bonds. The latter is a perfectly healthy expression of mourning for most individuals that encourages a subjective sense of the other's ongoing presence. But those who are mired in chronic grief or exhibiting features of a preoccupied response to loss should engage in illusory conversations with the deceased only insofar as doing so helps to confront reality. If not careful, enacting this type of ritual may tempt the bereaved to lose focus and carry on conversing with the dead as if present, an expression of grief work that may already be in abundance.

Searching rituals: Confirming physical absence

Just as the child instinctively knows to cry and smile in order to summon the caregiver's presence, the emergence of locomotive capabilities in the first twelve months brings with it a natural impulse to go search for attachment figures upon separation. Independent exploration is inhibited in an effort to focus attention on resuming proximity to the caregiver if time and space apart are beyond what is tolerable. These attachment behaviors are activated with equal ferocity after a loss, and John Bowlby (1963, 1980) argued that *they must be acted on consciously in order to facilitate a healthy course of mourning*. This fits well with Freud's (1917) observation that the bereaved will continue to direct psychic energy outward in search of the lost relationship, but only upon repeated failures to connect with someone who is no longer "out there" will acceptance of absence settle in. Only then will they pull back from efforts to find the attachment figure and mourn the finality of what death has taken away.

It is not uncommon for the bereaved to find themselves unconsciously compelled to search for the dead without being aware of the underlying meaning of their behavior. This impulse may play out in repetitive and unproductive ways that only stall the mourning process: a surreptitious wish to converse again with the deceased inspires a habitual pattern of calling their phone number and listening to the outgoing message; time is squandered taking alternate routes home that pass by where a loved one once lived; the bereaved establish new relationships with individuals who are eerily alike whoever had died; patterns of interaction once enjoyed with the deceased are recreated with others in a defensive attempt to ward off conscious awareness of anything having changed. The search party persists without clarifying whom they are looking for or what they expect to find.

One's subjective experience of loss and mourning has always been encumbered by nagging disbelief about the finality of death. It is for this reason that many grief rituals around the world center on actively seeking out confirmation of the deceased's absence. The Ifugao, an indigenous people on the island of Luzon in the Philippines, practice unique burial rituals that leave nothing to be doubted. Between death and interment of the body, an extended wake of at least three days allows for mourning and celebration of the deceased's life. But this liminal phase of mourning is also in place to ensure that the deceased *is*, indeed, dead. The corpse is seated in a chair near the family's house while a small cadre of women keep vigil. The Ifugao people believe that the soul may intermittently escape the body only to return within a short period of time. And so the women cry and shake the body repeatedly for three days to confirm that the deceased is truly gone before proceeding to burial and accepting that the soul has departed (Willcox, 1912).

The Ifugao are not the only peoples whose rituals center on corporeal interactions in order to confirm death. It is also customary in Japanese culture for the family to hold an overnight vigil over the body of the dead, an *otsuya*, a few days after death to confirm that they have passed. Family members are then expected to witness the corpse being slid into a cremation chamber, after which they will pick the bones out of ashes and place them into an urn (Valentine, 2010). And in rural areas of Haiti, where much of the population believe in voodoo and voodoo curses, there is concern that the dead may become reanimated as a zombie and bring about mental illness, viral infections, and tragic accidents. To combat these fears, autopsies are sometimes performed to verify that death has actually arrived, and many believe it is imperative to bury the dead beneath the ground, where they cannot harm the living (Rey & Stepick, 2013).

The Irish wake, with its customs of visitation and an open casket, originated in Ireland during the early twentieth century to make certain that the deceased had actually died before they were buried. Prominent use of pewter glassware at that time introduced risk of lead poisoning, which gave rise to concerns that a resulting catatonic state would give the false impression of death. Thus, the open-casket wake came to be as a means to confirm the reality of death and ensure that the living was not being buried alive (Grainger, 1998).

While some customs allow for brief contact with the corpse during a wake or funeral, many will neither have access to these funeral rites nor desire tactile encounters with the dead. If interaction with the body is not a viable option, what symbols can be used to confirm death, change, and the passing of time? Personal grief rituals can gravitate towards visiting *places* the deceased regularly frequented (the "where" of the ritual) to confirm that their presence no longer resides where it once did. In lieu of approaching the empty vessel of the body which the dead no longer inhabit, a physical space once occupied by the deceased can be approached with conscious willingness to process the pain of their loved one's absence. These searching rituals are, in a sense, designed to fail! The bereaved facilitates healthy mourning by looking for the deceased attachment figure in old haunts where they once were for the sole purpose of *not* finding them.

Jocelyn's dream, described at the beginning of this chapter, can be interpreted as a simple wish fulfillment: She and her father could continue to collaborate on household projects together just as they always had, and her father could still be found standing at his workbench as reliably as ever. While asleep, her mind carried on pursuing her father's proximity in protest against the passing of time she awoke to every morning. Jocelyn's waking thoughts and behaviors complemented this fanciful chase with a fearful evasion of his absence in the home. Jocelyn worked long hours away at her job. She skirted around conversations with her mother. When she was in the house, she hid in her bedroom and passed the time under a spell of sleep, eschewing the empty rooms her father once frequented.

Most strikingly, Jocelyn ceased spending time in the garage, where her father's tools remained idle. She told me early in our work together, "I don't want to see that he's not standing there." Home repair and woodworking had been her favorite pastimes since childhood when her father began teaching her the basics of how to swing a hammer or use a level. They forged a deep bond helping each other in the garage with whatever project required attention over the years. But since his death, Jocelyn avoided the garage altogether. Neglected household projects began to accumulate: a broken leg of a dining room chair collected dust in the attic, loose doorknobs made it difficult to open closets, a new ceiling fan was left uninstalled in the corner of the living room. She genuinely wanted to re-engage in her hobby, but she was afraid to confront the reality that her father would no longer be at her side.

Jocelyn and I began exploring how she could create a personal grief ritual that led her back to the garage, to dwell in that space and let her father's absence sink in. In theory, she would go searching for him with conscious intention, knowing she would not find him standing there, waiting for her. Jocelyn reserved an hour to explore the workbench for the first time since her father died, and she made a point to hold the tools in her hands as she wandered about, recalling the numerous repairs they had made to the ceiling, the electrical sockets, and the shelves that held tiny compartments for various nails and screws. In subsequent visits to the garage, Jocelyn invited her mother to join in. She recounted the stillness of the room, how its silence permeated her thoughts. After the most intense feelings of grief subsided, she and her mother spontaneously augmented the ritual with what would become an ongoing tradition: They would sit in the garage together, enjoy a beer, and regale each other with their favorite stories of living with a man who spent more time at his workbench than in any other room of the house.

Searching rituals like the one Jocelyn created hinge on *revisiting old haunts* where the deceased spent much time and could regularly be found while alive. A room where the deceased often dwelled is a common setting for such rituals, but the bereaved frequently yearn to step out of their homes, away from their day-to-day lives, and demarcate a sacred space in nature or on street corners where the ritual can be performed. The search party may be best dispatched by walking the aisles of the deceased's favorite bookstore, enjoying a coffee at a café they treasured, or meandering through a nature preserve where they used to linger. A notably different type of searching ritual can encourage the bereaved to return to locations where a singular fond memory or event of special significance occurred. The bereaved may even gravitate towards visiting the very sight where their loved one died.

While working with a man whose partner died in a bicycling accident after being hit by a car, I learned of an annual event called the Ride of Silence. Every third Wednesday evening in May, communities of cyclists in metropolitan cities across the United States honor fellow cyclists who lost their lives as a result of car accidents. They ride together along a path highlighted by locations where such deaths recently happened. The Ride of Silence aims to draw greater attention to the shocking number of bicycling fatalities that occur in cities with congested traffic. Cyclists are asked to remain silent as they bike from one site to the next, stopping along the route at each location to pause and mourn together. I have gathered that the Ride of Silence serves as a meaningful grief ritual with a profoundly deep function: to act on the instinct to search for the deceased and confirm the reality of their death by visiting the very spot where they died. I was not surprised to hear that the bicyclists grow sad and mournful as they pause to contemplate each of these losses in their community. Seeing as how complicated bereavement can stem from a failure to integrate awareness of the circumstances of where and how a death occurred, the Ride of Silence exemplifies how to incorporate important locations into grief rituals that facilitate deeper acceptance of loss.

A woman I once provided therapy to, Fiona, sought me out after her husband, a construction worker, accidentally fell to his death while doing a roofing project. It was a large commercial building tucked away in a wooded area away from the city. During the intake appointment, she revealed that she had been frequently distracted by what she felt was a bizarre and illogical thought that her husband was still lying beside the building or walking around in the nearby forest preserve. Even within her fantasies, Fiona was searching for her husband in a primitive and intuitive effort to resume proximity. She and I designed a onetime ritual in which she visited the spot where he died. As was planned, Fiona stayed for a significant stretch of time until feelings of upset arose and subsided (whenever creating this type of personal grief ritual with a client who has been avoiding a particular stimulus, including a location, I find it crucial to lean upon research on exposure therapy that observes how the individual must remain engaged in the previously avoided situation and resist the urge to flee, lest an avoidant response be reinforced further). I was pleased to hear that, following the performance of this ritual, Fiona's fantasy about searching for her husband no longer preoccupied her mind.

Releasing the soul and saying goodbye

The deceased's body, a once-useful, now-empty shell, is fated to lie in repose on earth, interred underground or dispersed in ashes across the land, but the soul's ultimate destination is not so certain. A survey of various worldviews offers up disparate beliefs about where the immaterial residue of life is bound to settle. Secularists and stoics assert that death amounts to no more than a redistribution of matter, including those substrates of the brain where one's soul must reside, back into the earth. Spiritual views provide reassurance that one's spirit will ascend into an afterworld fully intact, recognizable to loved ones with whom they hope to reunite.

Wherever one's beliefs lie, grief rituals throughout history and from all corners of the world have been designed with the express purpose of liberating the soul from its earthly dwellings and aiding in the transition from one plane of existence to the next. Whether looking to the ancient Egyptians, the Vikings that roamed northern Europe a thousand years ago, or Hindu traditions practiced in India and across the globe today, the ubiquity of this type of ritual speaks volumes to its value in the mourning process. But the dead are not the sole benefactors. As the living participate in efforts to release the soul into the afterlife, they are afforded a proper goodbye, a formal and resolute sendoff that helps relinquish earthly ties.

In a remote corner of China, the people of the Sanyuan Village, an amalgam of ten villages all located near the Dahong River Valley, participate in a sequence of multifaceted rituals that facilitate the deceased's peaceful departure. Once an elder is near death, kin are summoned and expected to be present to gather near the dying in their final days. Descendants from the village take shifts keeping vigil over the dying individual so that, before their final breath, they can be moved to a chair in the bedroom that faces the door. All the dying person's kin are to kneel around the chair while extended family remain standing and encircle the group. The eldest son is then expected to hold the dying family member upright. This is the precise moment when final words and farewells are to be spoken, a process the people of Sanyuan Village call *songzhong*, which means to send off the dying (Chen, 2000).

Chen (2000) explains that, within the Sanyuan Village, "to die in bed is considered harmful because the soul of the newly deceased cannot easily leave the bed due to a mosquito net usually emplaced all the year round, which would capture the soul of the deceased" (p. 70). Kin will still engage in more rituals designed to further facilitate transition into the afterlife and to drive away evil spirits and ghosts that otherwise threaten to haunt surviving family members and inflict illness, death, and other misfortunes. The body is placed on a wooden board in the home and readied for *mahang*, best translated as *ritually washing the deceased*. Kin's clothing, typically those of a son, are soaked in boiled water infused with eucalyptus leaves before being used to clean the body. The deceased is then dressed in clothes reserved for burial ahead of time, called *shouyi* (Birx, 2006). This ritualistic washing is believed to drive away evil spirits attached to the body while also granting the deceased the right to be accepted into the afterlife by their ancestors.

Many cultures bury their dead with cherished and valuable items to aid the soul in its journey. The ancient Egyptians felt compelled to bury their deceased with food, ritual money, and other talismans to facilitate the soul's travels through the spirit world. An image of the female god Nut, who was believed to protect and carry the dead to the afterlife, was etched into the bottom of a coffin. Such themes are teeming throughout ancient Greek burial practices and mythology as well. Charon, ferryman of Hades, was to be paid a fee if one wished to cross the river Styx. As follows, the ancient Greeks routinely placed coins in the mouth or over the eyes of their dead to pay Charon's toll.

Several of these practices persist today. The Zulu people of South Africa and Taoists across Asia provide the deceased with supplies necessary to sustain the soul through its voyage, including rice and other foods, money, and a flashlight to illuminate their path. Sanyuan villagers immediately initiate *Daotou fuzi* after a death, the burning of money in order to "provide the deceased with traveling expenses on the way to the world of the dead" (Chen, 2000, p. 71). Japanese Buddhists today bury the dead wearing sandals and accompanied by six gold coins, the fee sufficient to cross the Sanzu River on the way to the afterlife. It is also tradition in Japanese burials to place a dagger on the dead person's chest, a samurai-era custom designed to fend off evil spirits (*mamono*) along the way.

The rituals and customs described prior rest on the presumption that the soul is naturally pulled to exit this world, that it will ascend into the afterlife if only given safe passage. Conversely, a host of cultural death rites and rituals is predicated on a belief that the soul remains in limbo after death, lingering on earth to perturb the living if not persuaded to leave. Robert Hertz's (1960) classic analysis of the cultural practice of *secondary burials* captures the essence of such concerns. However grief-stricken those in mourning may be, they wait in eager anticipation for the buried corpse to eventually rot and decompose. To unearth the corpse after its initial interment and find that the body has decayed is cause for great relief; the subsequent burial of what remains offers reassurance that death has truly arrived and that malevolent ghosts will no longer burden or threaten harm unto the living.

The physical deconstruction of the corpse is taken as confirmation that the soul has also gone through a similar transformation in readying itself to depart from the world of the living. So too does the earthbound mourner undergo a metamorphosis of their own as they traverse through mourning and arrive at definitive acceptance of death and loss. Thus, Hertz demonstrated a keen appreciation for the symbolic relationship that binds the corpse, the soul, and the mourner together in parallel processes of transcendence, saying:

> To make a material object or living being pass from this world to the next, to free or create the soul, it must be destroyed. . . . As the visible object vanishes it is reconstructed in the beyond, transformed to a greater or lesser degree.
>
> (p. 46)

He added, "Death is fully consummated only when decomposition has ended; only then does the deceased cease to belong to this world so as to enter another life" (p. 47).

Not all cultural grief rituals find the bereaved rendered entirely passive, merely waiting for time to proceed as it will. Many cultures intentionally use loud noises to actively drive away bad spirits and prevent the dead from staying in the world of the living for too long. In the Sanyuan Village, these rituals occur immediately upon the dying person's last breath. Kin burst into a cacophony of wailing cries – this is primarily done by women – and ignite firecrackers to scare away ghosts thought to be wandering in the home and threatening harm if left undisturbed. And the Berawan people of Borneo deploy similar tactics to encourage the deceased spirit's departure. Their rituals consist of two major ceremonies, the first of which concludes by placing the corpse in a simple wooden coffin within a graveyard. After sufficient time has passed, anywhere from eight months to five years, the bones are then cleaned and transferred to their final resting place . . . but the dead have not completed their transition just yet. The Berawan believe that the spiritual component of the human, what they call the *telanak*, must be encouraged to embark on its journey to the land of the dead; this is facilitated by the singing of death songs as women perform dramatic dirges amid tearful sobbing (Metcalf & Huntington, 1991). Unlike the quietude of searching rituals that bask in the absence of noise to confirm that the deceased is no longer present, the production of loud noise serves as a catalyst that propels the dead into the next world.

In Japanese culture, it is believed that the deceased's spirit will ascend to the afterlife on the forty-ninth day after death. Just as the deceased must wander aimlessly in an intermediary holding pattern, neither alive on earth nor having begun their journey to the world of the dead, the living wait patiently in this liminal phase of mourning. When at last the forty-ninth day arrives and the funeral ceremonies begin, the ritual of *kaimyo* encourages the living to assign the deceased a new name. This is done so as to prevent the spirit from returning to the world of the living should they hear the bereaved utter their earthly name (Swarts, 2001).

One cannot help but wonder if these rituals, with their uniform anxiety about the soul lingering too long after death, crop up in distant corners of the world because of something ubiquitous about the beleaguered psyche in mourning. Perhaps the greatest threat lies not in the deceased's spirit hesitating to move on but in the bereaved hesitating to accept loss, relinquish old ties, and get on with life. Ghosts haunt him only insofar as he holds too tight to an invisible presence that must be released. And so rituals have evolved to goad the bereaved into actively letting go and pushing the dead away by paying the gatekeepers to the afterlife, creating noxious noises, and assigning the dead new names. The individual who creates their own personal grief ritual can choose how they would like to actively renounce their physical bond with the deceased in the most meaningful manner. A variety of symbolic items and actions may do. But for some, they need look no further than nature and the elements around them – fire, water, air, and earth – for tangible symbols of the transformation, movement, and release they so desire.

Rituals that incorporate the elements of nature: Fire

Humankind has long relied upon cremation as an alternative to interment of the body in a coffin, casket, or shroud, but its exact origins are uncertain. In 1968, a surprising discovery was made near Lake Mungo of New South Wales in Australia: the charred remains of a woman thought to have lived 42,000 years ago! What's striking is that the *Mungo Lady*, as she was affectionately named, was most certainly mourned in a ritualistic fashion, as evidenced by signs that her body was cremated, her bones were crushed, and then the remains were burned again before they were ultimately buried.

Various civilizations throughout history have resorted to this type of funeral rite. The custom ebbed and flowed in preference and frequency of use during the rise and fall of both the ancient Greek and ancient Roman empires. Literary sources attest to as much: In Homer's *Iliad*, we find an account of Patroclus's body being burned on a funeral pyre and subsequently buried, often regarded as the earliest written description of cremation. But with the advent of Christianity and its belief in the resurrection of the body, cremation fell largely out of practice throughout Europe by the fifth century and was, at various times, forbidden by law. The ancient Egyptians had also banned the practice, as it was believed that the soul could not transform into a new form and migrate to the afterlife if the body were reduced to ash. Many centuries later, late-nineteenth-century Europe once more saw a resurgence of cremation that has carried on unabated to this day.

A great many cultures have continued to find meaning in the use of cremation to pave a path upon which the soul can be liberated. During the age of the Vikings, spanning some three hundred years between the eighth and eleventh centuries AD, cremation was used regularly to mourn the dead, typically conducted on a funeral pyre consisting of a large quantity of timber, where the dead were burned along with personal objects to facilitate their passage to the afterlife in Valhalla. The remaining ashes would then be buried under a pile of rocks arranged in the shape of a ship, symbolizing the importance of sailing in Viking culture and the assumed role that these vessels played in helping the dead journey to Valhalla (Dougherty, 2014).

On the Indonesian island of Bali, cremation is believed to free the soul and release it into the afterlife. These Balinese ceremonies are not only considered a sacred duty but have also proven to be a celebratory social event. As Miguel Covarrubias (1937) wrote in his book *Island of Bali*, "Strange as it seems, it is in their cremation ceremonies that the Balinese have their greatest fun" (p. 325).

Hindu death rites, as practiced in Nepal and India, date back to approximately 500 BC and have long revolved around ritual cremation. The purpose of all Hindu death rites, or *sraddhas*, is to liberate the soul of the deceased and facilitate their transition towards joining the ancestors in the afterlife. Time is also allocated for the family to mourn, pay respects, and say goodbye to their loved ones (Hopkins, 1992). Dr. Vasudha Narayanan, in an interview with Beliefnet (2003), explained:

> Rituals give us a way of cathartically dealing with our grief. Every one of the rituals within the Hindu ceremonies is a reality check to help us confront our grief, interact with it, accept it and keep going on – both in life and spiritually.

Once a person has died, their body is purified through bathing and is dressed in new clothes. An oil lamp may then be placed near the body and left to burn for a period of three days following the death. Next, the body is transported to the site of the cremation ground and laid upon a funeral pyre prepared with lavish offerings of sandalwood and saffron covered in ghee to increase flammability. The chief mourner (either the eldest son, brother, or father of the deceased) walks around the body three times while sprinkling sacred water on the body and then uses a torch to ignite one section of wood at a time until flames have encircled the pyre. It is at this point that a traditional thirteen-day mourning period begins for the family. The use of fire in the oil candles is thought to evoke Brahma, the divine god of Hinduism represented by the breath of all living things and of fire. The cremation process itself symbolizes Brahma releasing the soul of the deceased to the world of the ancestors. On the twelfth day after death, a feast is held to commemorate the dead, who will continue to be remembered during successive monthly *sraddha* celebrations of the ancestors (Cush et al., 2008).

Meaningful interactions with the body are pivotal in many cultures' efforts to relinquish the soul, bid farewell, and confirm absence. But the bereaved individual may not have access to such corporeal rituals. If she cannot hold a dying family member up to a doorway as they take their last breath, or if he cannot unearth the remains and rebury them to confirm that the body has perished, or if she cannot destroy the empty vessel of flesh and bones with fire, one can set up alternate symbols to be relinquished, knocked down, or even obliterated. Personal grief rituals *can be designed around abstract representations of the deceased* that, in symbolic gestures, give the bereaved something to let go of and say goodbye to. This type of substitute for the body regularly centers on inanimate objects to be renounced: ashes, personal possessions, property, balloons, etc. The bereaved may also wish to jettison these representations of the dead in meaningful locations. Nature, in all its forms, regularly provides the desired background. To stand among elements of water, air, and earth is to surround oneself with poignant reminders of the transience in all things. The cadence of growth and decay pulls organic life back into the waves, the wind, and the soil beneath one's feet.

The element of fire tends to be used in efforts to let go with a more decidedly destructive force, though not necessarily out of hostility or vindictiveness. It is simply a matter of initiating immediate change and alteration that one can gaze upon as it occurs. To burn a symbol of the dead and watch it be swallowed by flames is to observe spontaneous transformation in action: An object in one form immediately comes to assume another. Solid matter morphs into smoke and ash that dissipates upwards, just as a life may remold into its spiritual essence before reaching for the heavens.

Hal was a young man whose husband, Ian, died after many grueling years fighting cancer. Hal could not shake the feeling that he was still his husband's "protector" even after death. He had nursed Ian through years of illness, painful treatments, and round after round of remission and relapse. His very sense of self revolved around being at his husband's side. When Ian finally lost his fight, and with it his life, Hal was aimless and uncertain about what to do with himself moving forward.

Hal clung to his role as Ian's "protector" with one futile pursuit after another. He attempted to file a medical malpractice suit against the doctors that worked with Ian towards the end but was told he had no case. He tried in vain to patch up Ian's estranged relationship with his family members, many of whom did not accept Ian because of his sexuality; they remained unswayed by Hal's pleas to let him tell them of the good and kind person Ian was and that the love they had for each was real. Of greatest upset was the troubled relationship Ian had with his own father, who had abused him mercilessly as a child. Hal felt powerless. He could not turn back the clock to provide any additional care or to safeguard Ian from further heartbreak.

After a year into his therapy with me, Hal divulged something he had been feeling self-conscious about: He wished to leave the past behind him and move forward with his life. He wanted to date again. He wanted to move out of the apartment in which Ian had spent his last days, ultimately dying in their living room. He wanted to find a new job, in a new city perhaps. But he still felt held back by a sense of duty to his husband. I offered my simple observation that he would benefit from letting go of that role which once made sense, to which he responded, "I want to, but I don't know how to . . ." He stopped to motion as if pushing something away and said, "get away from it." I asked Hal if he would find meaning in getting rid of any of Ian's possessions that he was still holding on to or any inanimate objects that symbolized the caretaker role that continued to grip him. Hal pondered over this for a while and then shared that in all his ventures to hospitals, lawyers' offices, and Ian's family, he had been carrying around an urn with his partner's ashes.

Because Ian's family disapproved of their marriage, Hal was never invited to the funeral. He had never had a proper chance to say goodbye in any meaningful fashion. To remedy this, Hal ultimately decided to reserve time for a personal grief ritual during which he would spread the majority of Ian's ashes. I pressed him to think about any meaningful locations where he would like to do so, and he immediately brought to mind the park along the Chicago River where they had met for their first date many years ago. He planned to go on a day when the weather resembled that of their first meeting. It was a late-spring afternoon, still cool enough to feel the brisk wind coming off the water but warm enough to feel the sun on his face heralding warmer months ahead. Ian always enjoyed paddling down the river in a kayak with his husband to unwind and take in some sightseeing. Hal decided to rent a kayak for himself and take in the nature and soaring architecture of downtown like they once did together before spreading Ian's ashes into the river. But before completing this ritual, he brought along an additional item to release: a painstaking journal entry Ian had written in an imaginary conversation with his father to express the lifetime of pain his father's abuse had caused. He burned the letter and found immense joy in watching the embers die and fall into the river before spreading Ian's ashes. For Hal, this ritual represented a significant release from a cruel world that had pained his husband greatly. At the same time, the ritual's location symbolized the love that his husband found in their union, his hope that Ian would forever have that love with him wherever he now was, and Hal's own sense of liberation from the protector role that no longer served either of them.

Rituals that incorporate the elements of nature: Water

The personal grief ritual that Hal designed, though centered on ash and fire, also evidenced how water can be incorporated into expressions of grief and mourning that confirm absence. If fire pulls the soul up towards the heavens, bodies of water gently carry it out with the tide, away from the shore of the living. Furthermore, many cultures previously described find great meaning in the inherent symbolism of water as that which cleanses the old and ushers in fresh beginnings: Bathing the body serves to wash away residue from this life and provide a direct, hands-on confrontation with what has come to pass.

The Hindu ritual of *sapindikarana*, best translated as *grouping together*, uses water to represent the soul being merged with those of the forefathers and received into the world of ancestors, the *pitrlaka*. On the twelfth day following a death, Brahmana priests are invited to partake in a memorial service during which four vessels of water are mixed, one for the deceased's *preta* and one for each of the three generations of forefathers that had preceded, the *pitrs*. As the vessels of water are mixed together, the names of the *pitrs* are spoken by the priest and their unification is confirmed. It is believed that the *preta* body of the deceased will become a ghost and be blocked from the *pitrloka* if these rituals are not performed. Thus, the completion of this water-based ritual marks a definitive end to the deceased's earthly journeys (Knipe, 1977).

I have long suspected that grief rituals which involve submersion into water appeal to a quiet belief that many hold dear in their hearts: In death, the essence of a living being is dissolved back into an oceanic and undifferentiated state, free from concerns of having to navigate a world in which one all too often feels separate and alone. The bereaved, still traversing their own sojourn through life, can incorporate the symbolism of water into personal grief rituals to help them reflect upon how the deceased, upon departing, have been absorbed into the larger whole of what lies beyond.

Rituals that incorporate the elements of nature: Air

In Gabriel Garcia Marquez's masterpiece *One Hundred Years of Solitude*, a character by the name of Remedios the Beauty spontaneously ascends skyward to her death, forever out of sight to those who looked upon her loveliness with awe and adoration. She seemed to have been summoned by the heavens in a haunting and ethereal exit. This fictional passage feels all too real to anyone who has watched a loved one float further and further out of view as they depart from the world. Thus, air, sky, and wind provide valuable metaphors by which to comprehend the reality of loss and absence, of a life having been swept away by some force of nature beyond us. Just as the whims of the wind whisk away its object with no warning, so too does death indiscriminately pluck its prey from the earth below. And when the bereaved speaks of those he has lost, he instinctively looks up towards the sky; the dead, it seems, reside eternally overhead in the stars and in our minds.

Tibetan Buddhists, in both Mongolia and Tibet, believe in the transmigration of the spirit after death. The soul is thought to move on, upward, while the shell of the body remains bound to earth, rendered no more than an empty vessel. As follows, burial of the corpse is deemed a hollow gesture. Approximately 80 percent choose instead to dispose of the dead by performing a meaningful ritual in practice for thousands of years: the *sky burial*. So as to ease the spirit's transition, the deceased's bodily remains are placed on a mountaintop, where they are to be exposed to the elements of nature and to carrion, including vultures, who will consume the flesh and entrails and proceed to lift the soul up into the sky. After many days have passed, the bereaved eventually return to discover that the bones have been picked clean (Goss & Klass, 1997; Joyce & Williamson, 2003). Sky rituals provide one of the most blunt methods by which to confirm absence. But this practice is only available and/or desirable to a select few in the world. In what other ways might air and sky be incorporated into personal grief rituals that facilitate more profound acceptance of death?

Rick, discussed at the beginning of the chapter, dreamed of spending a mundane Wednesday afternoon getting lunch with his dear friend Nia at their favorite diner just as they had done for years. Despite its quotidian content, this dream perfectly captured Rick's experience of grief since Nia died suddenly from a brain aneurysm seven months prior. He was lonely and missed his lifelong friend's consistent company. Furthermore, Rick was hesitant to take the edge off his solitude by forging new relationships or strengthening those he already had. He remained withdrawn in quiet protest against the loss of his best friend.

Rick and Nia had lived together as roommates in Milwaukee for eleven years. Rick eventually moved back to Chicago a few years prior to her tragic death, but despite the distance, they maintained frequent contact and saw each other at least a few times every month. Rick would occasionally drive all the way up to Milwaukee on an errant Wednesday afternoon just to keep up the tradition of grabbing lunch together at their old haunt, sometimes spending the night on the couch in the apartment they once shared, where Nia still lived. As he no longer had any reason to drive up north to eat at the diner or stay in their old apartment, his day-to-day life in Chicago was devoid of any reminders of the past he enjoyed with his friend. Rick assumed this would be to his benefit, as he feared that reminiscence would only evoke painful nostalgia. But alas, it became increasingly apparent that he was hiding from confrontations with reality. Loneliness persisted, and though he wanted to quell this pain in earnest, opening himself to new friendships was felt to be an admission of defeat, a white flag signaling acceptance of the uncomfortable truth that he would never again retrieve the company of his best friend.

One day, while discussing his practice of Buddhism, Rick referenced a traditional Buddhist ritual he had always been fond of that involved throwing sand into water, a symbolic gesture of letting go. I asked him if he wanted to enact this type of ritual, but specifically for the sake of confronting the loss of his friend. He immediately declined and opted instead to release balloons into the air, saying he and Nia had always joked about how "flighty" she could be. Without prompting of any kind, Rick knew exactly where he wanted to carry this out. He quickly made plans to drive up to Milwaukee on a Wednesday afternoon and send purple balloons – purple was her favorite color – careening into the clouds from two important locations: the diner and their apartment. Rick returned to therapy the following week and reported that the experience turned out to be quite evocative. Releasing a symbolic representation of Nia into the air left him with a visceral sense that he had been holding on to her too tightly. And as he sailed the purple balloons out of sight into an overcast sky, he noticed an involuntary nod, an embodied acknowledgment that he would need to find a new friend with whom he could grab lunch when feeling lonely.

Incorporating the elements of nature: Relinquishing earthly ties

Carina's husband of over forty years, Leonard, died after three years of battling leukemia. Much of his fight was waged in their home during his final year. As he grew increasingly feeble, Carina's life became enveloped in his care. She was his cook, his in-home nurse who administered his drugs, his personal chauffeur, his tailor, laundress, seamstress, and more. It was a daily grind. She was sad and confused and exhausted . . . and she loved it. Carina would have been happy to shoulder the burden of her husband's ill health for the rest of her days. But when Leonard's life finally expired, all that was left of her husband was his stuff: his clothes, his books, mementoes from a lifetime of travels, the many musical instruments he played, and box after box filled with medical supplies. These things were no longer of any use. And the home they lived in for four decades was now too big for her alone, a mere storehouse for her past life with Leonard that she could not keep up on her own. Carina knew that it was time to relocate. It was time to enjoy her retirement and the life that remained, but she was immobilized. She could not let go. The foundation of her life with Leonard, their home and all his belongings, was firmly planted in the ground. Though she genuinely wished to move forward, Carina could not bring herself to rip out the roots.

The elements of fire, air, and water are in perpetual motion. Flames sway back and forth in a hypnotizing dance. The waves of the sea undulate on the horizon. A gale of wind pivots this way and that as it blows with tremendous force. Earth, on the other hand, errs towards stillness. The soil we tread upon settles and becomes more compact over time. And so the element of earth itself becomes a fitting metaphor for those deeply entrenched in a course of mourning that does not seem to budge. It is often the inanimate earthly possessions one holds on to, both big and small, that weigh heavy and pin them to the ground. Many individuals like Carina struggle to move forward because they will not let go of the things that represent the dead, be it a shirt or a house. Those cultures who bury the dead with their possessions beneath the surface, beyond reach, are acting on the imperative to relinquish that which is no longer of use aboveground.

Australian Aborigines' rituals hinge upon a similar imperative to drive the spirit off the land away from previous attachments to the home so as to ensure their safe passage into the afterlife, what they refer to as *the Dreamtime*. One of their most common rites involves a smoking ceremony in which the bereaved gather in the deceased person's home and smolder native plants to ward off bad spirits. Plumes of smoke billow over personal belongings and throughout corners of the house where they spent the majority of their time, including the very spot where they died. Yet another ritual involves extracting ocher deposits from clay in the ground and applying it as a paint on all living spaces once inhabited by the deceased (McGrath & Phillips, 2008).

After spending months wandering alone through their old home, Carina knew the time had come to let go of her lot of land and move elsewhere. Her home felt both cluttered and poignantly empty, a collection of relics from the life she and Leonard once lived that now only made her sad. But she was afraid to part ways and confront her loss further, saying, "Once I get rid of all that stuff, it's gonna feel so much more real." Indeed, ridding one's space of the deceased's possessions often evokes a keen sense of their absence.

Carina and I developed a personal grief ritual in which she could let go of these earthly ties, however slowly. She brought in a few select items – old hats, dusty and torn books, leftover medical ointments – into successive therapy sessions and bade them farewell. As if speaking directly to Leonard, she said goodbye as she placed one item after another into a garbage basket in my office. Carina would later comment on the experience, saying, "Getting rid of all that stuff felt like a piece of my guts being cut out . . . but it's just stuff." Her confrontation with loss and absence was not wholesale. Carina decided to still hold on to a few select things near and dear to her memory of Leonard that she could carry with her into her new home. And when the house itself was sold, we agreed that it would be meaningful for her to walk through one last time alone to say goodbye.

On the heels of the three-year anniversary of Leonard's passing, Carina reported a dream that once again involved only her and Leonard. She vaguely recalled that they were having fun together, but the dream ended with Carina looking to Leonard and saying, "But you're dead." The reality of her husband's absence had finally set in, and I trusted that our work was complete.

References

Becker, E. (1973). *The denial of death*. Free Press Paperbacks.

Beliefnet. (2003, February). *Hindu rituals for death and grief*. www.beliefnet.com/faiths/hinduism/2003/02/hindu-rituals-for-death-and-grief.aspx

Birx, H. J. (2006). *Encyclopedia of anthropology*. SAGE Publications.

Bonetti, R. (2019). Living coffins and death among the Ga of Ghana. In H. Selin & R. M. Rakoff (Eds.), *Death across cultures: Death and dying in non-western cultures* (Vol. 9, pp. 167–192). Springer Publishing Company.

Bowlby, J. (1963). Pathological mourning and childhood mourning. *Journal of the American Psychoanalytic Association, 11*, 500–541.

Bowlby, J. (1980). *Attachment and loss: Vol. 3. Loss: Sadness and depression*. Basic Books.

Chen, G. (2000). *Death rituals in a Chinese village: An old tradition in contemporary social context* (Publication No. 9971525) [Doctoral dissertation, The Ohio State University]. ProQuest Dissertations Publishing.

Covarrubias, M. (1937). *Island of Bali*. Alfred A. Knopf.

Cush, D., Robinson, C., & York, M. (2008). *Encyclopedia of Hinduism*. Routledge.

Dougherty, M. J. (2014). *Vikings: A dark history of the Norse people*. New Holland Publishers.

Freud, S. (1917). Mourning and melancholia. *Standard Edition, 14*, 243–258. Hogarth Press.

Freud, S. (1926). Inhibitions, symptoms, and anxiety. *Standard Edition, 20*, 75–174. Hogarth Press.

Goss, R., & Klass, D. (1997). Tibetan Buddhism and the resolution of grief: The Bardo-thodol for the dying and the grieving. *Death Studies, 21*(4), 377–395.

Grainger, R. (1998). Let death be death: Lessons from the Irish wake. *Mortality, 3*(2), 129–141.

Hershberger, P. J., & Walsh, W. B. (1990). Multiple role involvements and the adjustment to conjugal bereavement: An exploratory study. *OMEGA – Journal of Death and Dying, 21*(2), 91–102.
Hertz, R. (1960). A contribution to the study of the collective representations of death. In R. Needham & C. Needham (Eds.), *Death and the right hand* (pp. 27–86). Free Press.
Hopkins, T. J. (1992). Hindu views of death and afterlife. In H. Obayashi (Ed.), *Death and afterlife: Perspectives of world religions* (pp. 143–155). Greenwood Press.
Joyce, K. A., & Williamson, J. B. (2003). Body recycling. In C. D. Bryant (Ed.), *Handbook of death & dying* (Vol. 2, pp. 775–785). Sage.
Kiong, T. C. (1993). The inheritance of the dead: Mortuary rituals among the Chinese in Singapore. *Southeast Asian Journal of Social Science, 21*(2), 130–158.
Knipe, D. M. (1977). Sapindikarana: The Hindu rate of entry into heaven. In F. E. Reynolds & E. Waugh (Eds.), *Religious encounters with death: Insights from the history and anthropology of religion* (pp. 111–124). Penn State University Press.
Levine, E. (1997). Jewish views and customs on death. In P. Laungani & W. Young (Eds.), *Death and bereavement across cultures* (pp. 98–130). Routledge.
McGrath, P., & Phillips, E. (2008). Insights on end-of-life ceremonial practices of Australian Aboriginal peoples. *Collegian, 15*(4), 125–133.
Metcalf, P., & Huntington, R. (1991). *Celebrations of death: The anthropology of mortuary ritual.* Cambridge University Press.
Nabokov, V. (1997). *Lolita.* Random House, Inc.
Rey, T., & Stepick, A. (2013). *Crossing the water and keeping the faith: Haitian religion in Miami.* NYU Press.
Saito, C. (2014). Engaging in grief ministry in multireligious contexts. *Pastoral Psychology, 63*(1), 105–112.
Stroebe, M., & Schut, H. (1999). The dual process model of coping with bereavement: Rationale and description. *Death Studies, 23*, 197–224.
Swarts, E. D. (2001). – *Kaimyo (Japanese Buddhist posthumous names) as indicators of social status* (Publication No. 3022582) [Doctoral dissertation, The Ohio State University]. ProQuest Dissertations Publishing.
Valentine, C. (2010). The role of the ancestral tradition in bereavement in contemporary Japanese society. *Mortality, 15*(4), 275–293.
Walker-Gillet, S. (2011). Death: Indigenous and western views. *Undergraduate Journal of Native Studies: Dbaajmowin, 1*, 83–102.
Willcox, C. D. W. (1912). *The head hunters of northern Luzon: From Ifugao to Kalinga, a ride through the mountains of northern Luzon.* Franklin Hudson Pub. Co.
Worden, J. W. (2008). *Grief counseling and grief therapy: A handbook for the mental health practitioner* (4th ed.). Springer Publishing Company.

Chapter 5

Expressing grief

Rituals that expand and limit emotional experiences of loss

Lucy was a thirty-one-year-old woman who came to psychotherapy one month after her father died of a long bout with non-Hodgkin's lymphoma. She had enjoyed a very supportive relationship with him. Lucy always felt understood, saying, "He and I were the same person." Unfailingly, her father conveyed great interest in her ambitious career goals as an educator; at the time of his death, Lucy was already climbing the ranks and impressing her superiors at a relatively young age. She was eager to seek out her father's guidance and regularly confided the details of her stress to him. He bolstered her esteem at times of frustration and doubt. He called her every day to check in and ask how she was doing. If she had an important meeting or job interview, he was the first to congratulate her successes with kind and encouraging words. I braced myself for what I figured would be a painful first meeting, and yet Lucy seemed to be doing well. She was moving forward with steadfast commitment to her career goals. She was embarking on her first venture into home ownership. When asked to describe her emotional response to her father's death, she calmly stated, "It's so sad, of course. I miss him, but it isn't crushing me or anything like that."

After three appointments, Lucy reduced the frequency of our meetings. She would begin sessions by flashing an energetic smile and launching into conversations about her recent breakup with her boyfriend, the relentless demands of work, and the disappointment of realizing the limits of what $300,000 will get you when buying a condominium in Chicago. I would slide in a question or two about her father and her grief, and she would respond with, "Just wish I could call him for advice," shrugging her shoulders in futility and continuing, "But I'm happy he taught me a lot while he was here." Lucy seemed to be doing . . . fine.

Grief: Too much or too little?

Loss will invariably inspire an emotional response. Myriad feelings have the potential to emerge from grief, and although most are marked by their noxious quality, some are innocuous or even downright pleasant. Be it sadness or

DOI: 10.4324/9781351204873-5

joy; anxiety, anger, or contentment; numb shock or an exhilarating sense of being moved; guilt, loneliness, or liberation, a distinct arrangement of emotions will bloom forth from within each individual's subjective experience of a loss. Where one person rages and shakes his fist at fate, another exhales a deep sigh of relief that a loved one no longer has to combat a progressive illness, and still another alternates between anguish-filled tears and gratitude for having had such a wonderful relationship that is painful to lose. The same individual may very well experience all of the above in quick succession. Each of these feelings is normative in and of itself, devoid of inherent complications. Indeed, an assortment of disparate emotions in concert with one another is the *sine qua non* of a self-restorative process of mourning.

Wherever the path of grief may lead, the journey often begins with shock. And this is a good thing. Muted disconnect is quite adaptive in the early throes of mourning, as it is not advisable to plumb the full depths of emotional pain immediately after a loss. A dulling of the senses barricades against emotional flooding. Shock conserves mental resources so that the bereaved can notify family members of the loss, make funeral arrangements, finalize end-of-life legal matters, and so on. Nonetheless, the stopgap of numbness must give way in due time and allow affect to trickle through. Grief must be felt. But the bereaved can certainly suffer from an excess of such. It is equally imperative that the bereaved not open the floodgates too wide or for too long lest she drown in a deluge of emotional pain. Thus, mourning provides no escape from the necessity of emotional response, a catch-22 in which the activation of feelings will surely burden the bereaved, but the evasion of such will inevitably weigh them down all the same.

All categories of complicated bereavement are marked by an unhealthy volume of emotional expression, be it surplus or shortfall. *Chronic grief* entails heightened emotional pain that does not abate over time. It manifests as intense yearning and an unremitting desire to maintain closeness with the deceased (Boelen & Klugkist, 2011). True, there is no consensus regarding how long mourning may persist before being deemed pathological and unduly protracted; grief and mourning about a particular loss will likely resurface intermittently throughout one's life. But the intensity of sorrow and pain should yield and ease over time, however slow and painstaking the pace may be. Chronic grief, however, continues to burst forth with steady force, unmitigated by time. Unrelenting emotional pain may even lead to the development of a full-blown psychological condition characterized by disruptive affect or anxiety, referred to as *exaggerated grief*. Otherwise, healthy expressions of sadness swell and crush the bereaved under the weight of depression. The occasional reprieve of happiness and goal-directed activity morphs into frenzied and euphoric pursuits of self-destructive pleasure amid a manic episode. The typical sting of anxiety festers and creates prolonged responses of shock and dread that incite panic attacks and symptoms of PTSD.

Whereas some instances of complicated bereavement are the product of excessive emotion, *delayed grief* occurs when emotions are tamped down and not adequately processed, only to rear their head after a significant amount of time has lapsed. Many bereaved individuals begin to seek out therapeutic services many years after a loss, when the depths of grief begin to pour out with an intensity that would suggest a loved one had died only a week prior. *Masked grief* also has its origins in scant expression of feelings, but its telltale sign is a lack of conscious awareness about the connection between symptoms of distress and the loss that had preceded. Grief registers in physiological discomforts and illnesses, such as tension headaches and ulcers and irritable bowel syndrome, compulsive behaviors, or intrusive emotional outbursts that seem unjustifiable to the bereaved and leave them confused. Despite Lucy's best efforts to carry herself with an air of nonchalance, her heartache could not be hidden away forever. True feelings of grief eventually broke through her defenses and revealed themselves in workplace stress and a growing sense of irritability and withdrawal from friends. For months after her father's passing, Lucy remained unaware of how these upsets had anything to do with one another.

This all poses a crucial question: What *is* the ideal quantity of emotional expression to secure a healthy course of mourning? Although difficult to pin down, the answer surely lies somewhere between the perils of excessive grief and the insidious trappings of insufficient venting; grief that is tethered too tight needs to be let loose, while unbridled shows of pain must be occasionally reined in. Each culture attempts to answer this question through the customs it prescribes. As discussed in Chapter 1, many cultures use rituals to facilitate expression of specific emotions regarding the deceased's absence. It is customary for Koreans to intentionally wail at various moments throughout the mourning process, including the moments immediately after death and during the funeral. These shows of sorrow and dedication to the deceased, what they call a *kok*, may also be used to convey guilt should the bereaved wrestle with concerns that a lack of pious action on their part may have contributed to the death (Lee, 1996).

Others' rituals err towards encouraging restraint and constriction. The Toraja people of Tana Toraja, like many southeast Asian cultures, value emotional control. They see intense grief as potentially harmful and permit only limited expression of sorrow through crying, wailing, and calling out to the dead while proximal to the corpse (Wellenkamp, 1991). Muslims also hold emotional restraint in high regard, as excessive lamentations are thought to be a disturbance to the dead (Kerrigan, 2017). And in highland Ecuador, indigenous beliefs in the power of negative emotions, including envy, to cause death motivate inhibition of their expression in mourning (Rosenblatt, 1997). Even the dynamics within a family can thwart emotional expression for select individuals, particularly those deemed to be *the strong one* (Worden, 2008). For instance, I have worked with numerous women in matriarchal family structures who have felt pressured to keep *their* grief in check so that others are permitted to let their guard down and mourn.

Given the universality of death, it is tempting to search for a ubiquitous experience of grief, some through line that highlights what grief feels like as well as the ideal amount of emotional expression required in order to mourn. But alas, we find no common denominator. Different cultures feel their losses differently from one another in both quantity and quality. So too does each individual differ in regard to what they feel and how much should come forth. The collective shows of solidarity provided by culture may or may not jibe with their emotional needs. The individual's subjective experience of grief is a moving target that culture often misses. One Korean individual may indeed benefit from regular acts of wailing to express intense sorrow and guilt, whereas the person standing at their side may already be overwhelmed with the intensity of his grief and would benefit more from opportunities to limit sorrow or to act on entirely different feelings of anger or joy. In those instances when cultural standards coax out excessive emotional expressions, restrict and muzzle what needs to be voiced, or encourage a specific feeling inauthentic to what the individual feels, personal grief rituals can facilitate a healthier outlet.

The attachment perspective: Is it beneficial to expand or limit expressions of grief?

Should the bereaved err towards maximizing emotional expression or minimizing it? Stroebe's dual process model (DPM) of coping with bereavement offers a helpful way to reconcile this tension. Loss-oriented and restoration-oriented stress both entail experiencing feelings related to grief, but where loss-oriented stress involves feelings of sadness, anger, and guilt specifically *about the loss of a meaningful relationship with the deceased*, restoration-oriented stress involves feelings pertaining more to secondary losses amid efforts to adjust to life after a death. According to Stroebe and Schut (1999), it is crucial for the bereaved to oscillate back and forth between these polarized emotional strains, confronting and coping with one while intentionally suppressing and avoiding the other for a time. Differing presentations of complicated bereavement are tied directly to a lack of such oscillation, with a heavy emphasis on one at the expense of neglecting the other. And therein lies the impediment to healthy mourning for many: consistently low or high emotional expression *about the deceased's absence*.

The one-size-fits-all solutions that cultural rituals offer run the risk of aggravating what is already lopsided for select members within the community. In such instances, personal grief rituals can help the bereaved design meaningful activities that right the ship and allow for a healthier balance of emotional expression about the dead. Perhaps an individual feels powerless but to emote with excessive intensity and frequency; participating in cultural rituals that facilitate greater emotional expression will only pour gasoline on the fire! Thus, creating a personalized approach that limits emotional expression and carves out time to manage secondary losses and stress will help him move forward in mourning. By contrast, if the individual's experience of grief is largely devoid of overt feeling about the deceased, cultural rituals that discourage loss-oriented stress will only tamp down emotional expression further. These individuals should consider implementing personal grief rituals that intentionally extract a more visceral emotional response so as to awaken critical grief work.

Some individuals, regardless of available rituals and the social values in which they are embedded, are destined to experience a dearth of feelings about a loss. This is particularly the case for those with a *dismissing attachment style*, who shy away from outward yearning and ruminations about the deceased. They may be quick to relinquish ties to the deceased under the pretense of moving on, and in doing so, they afford themselves inadequate time to process the pain inherent in letting go of a meaningful relationship. True to form, they will likely exhibit low reliance upon others for support and display minimal upset when family and friends are nearby. Such bottled-up emotions leave them vulnerable to delayed or masked variations of complicated grief. When emotion is acknowledged, it is limited to terse statements devoid of affective resonance, such as "It's sad" or "I've been a little angry ever since he died." These are examples of what William Worden (2008) means when he states that the bereaved need to do more than identify and articulate feelings: *The individual must experience their grief.* Naturally drawn towards an asymmetrical focus on restoration-oriented stress, those with a dismissing attachment style require rituals that evoke greater loss-oriented emotion about the deceased's absence.

Conversely, those with a preoccupied attachment style are susceptible to excessive loss-oriented emotional pain after a loss (Stroebe et al., 2005). Telltale signs include regular and intense displays of crying and painful yearning for the deceased, ruminative thoughts about the deceased, and an avoidance of activities or relationships unrelated to the deceased (Schenck et al., 2016). This constellation of symptoms regularly renders a chronic course of grief: Emotional expression does not extinguish itself, and behaviors focused entirely on the deceased only make the bereaved feel exponentially worse as they stew in perpetual mourning.

Intriguing research on complicated bereavement has used brain imaging techniques to illuminate why some bereaved individuals seek out activities that reliably make them ache. Behaviors associated with intense grief may, at first glance, seem like nonsensical compulsions that only stoke misery, such as looking at photos of the deceased for hours on end or repeatedly visiting a grave site and crying. Surprisingly, these expressions of sorrow and longing make complete sense once we delve deeper into the individual's multifaceted subjective experience. Brain images of the bereaved while engaging in such activities suggest that grief triggers conflicting emotions of pain and pleasure within the brain: While the pain network of the brain is active and motivating a retreat from noxious experiences, the reward centers of the brain are simultaneously motivating the bereaved to continually approach the agonizing experience of grief (O'Connor et al., 2008). For some individuals, their minds are in conflict about whether or not to continue expressing grief that, although self-reinforcing, routinely ushers in more distress!

Regardless of attachment style, those who find themselves mired in unrelenting grief will benefit from efforts to limit emotional expression. Such an assertion flies in the face of what many, laypeople and professionals alike, believe to be an indispensable part of mourning: Emotions must be expressed in full until expended. But striving to limit and contain grief is not tantamount to an outright bypass of feelings; rather, personal grief rituals can allocate circumscribed structures of time and space for metered emotional expression that prevents an endless outpouring of pain that would otherwise bleed into every facet of life and saturate the mourning process. Nonetheless, individuals with a preoccupied attachment style may struggle mightily to limit the expression of emotional pain once it is drawn out. They may benefit instead from rituals that sidestep sorrow that is specifically about the past (loss-oriented stress) and create an outlet for feelings of anger and joy about the restoration-oriented stresses that lie ahead.

And for those who require greater emotional expression, personal grief rituals should be designed with a focus on coaxing out loss-oriented affect. Opening the floodgates is rarely of concern for these individuals. Per the configurations of their personality and attachment style, defenses will naturally resume and tamp down feelings before they become excessive. In fact, any professional helping to design emotionally evocative rituals for a dismissing client may need to practice a bit of diplomacy and invite the client's thoughts about implementing specific parameters around its performance so that those who are resistant to emotional display do not run for the hills. It may be best for the ritual to provoke an emotional response for only five minutes or only within a specific location away from the home.

Opening the floodgates: Using activities to evoke and expand emotional expression about the deceased

Bereaved individuals require more than spoken language to truly experience grief. The beleaguered soul craves a visceral embodiment of all that is felt, and yet talk therapy all too often gets it wrong, reducing emotional expression to nothing more than the uttering of words to identify feeling states while sitting motionless. She lets out no more than, "I feel . . . sad" or "annoyed," "numb," or "angry." Full emotional experience, so crucial to the mourning process, gets lost in mere words and remains only partially processed. The Cartesian mind-body split, it seems, still prevails in the therapist's office.

Many cultural rituals, such as the reading of eulogies, aim to evoke a healthy emotional response among members of the community (Kunkel & Dennis, 2003). As helpful as invitations to cry and to laugh may be, they cast the bereaved into a passive role in which they do nothing but respond to another's emotional cues. Personal grief rituals can encourage a more active pursuit of emotional evocation, be it a wide range of sorrow, happiness, rage, guilt, and anxiety, or a singular emotion that needs to emerge and take shape amid mourning.

Let us return to the case of Lucy to explore how personal grief rituals can be centered on activities that evoke and expand emotional expression about the deceased. Lucy exhibited a consistent response to the dreaded question, "How does that make you feel?" She would always begin to give voice to feelings about her father's death only to quickly choke them back with a sharp, self-directed rebuke. She once described her grief as "pointless." Any expectation to cry or convey frustration in hopes of receiving support from others was, in her opinion, "manipulative." Emotional expression was felt to be inherently "selfish." It was no surprise, then, that Lucy had become withdrawn from her social life after her father died. She immersed herself deeply into work instead. When she did spend time with friends, the experience left her frustrated and disappointed. I could not help but notice a connection between the reason others were failing to give her what she wanted and her description of her relationship with her father: Her friends *didn't* understand her; "We *aren't* the same people," she'd say. Her friends seemed to have *no* interest in her career, and they certainly *were not* able to offer any sage advice. I, in turn, found myself pulled to ask her questions about her career and the interviews she was preparing for. Lucy, in turn, began giving me excited updates whenever we met for an appointment.

Christopher Hitchens once stated, "Something deemed unsayable is, sooner or later, bound to be said. And it may be said rather more heatedly as a result of it having been a taboo" (Hitchens et al., 2011, p. 9). Despite one's efforts to repress grief, feelings about a loss will gain expression one way or another, often through some distorted path of least resistance. Furthermore, as discussed in the previous chapter, the emotionally charged instinct to search for the deceased attachment figure will play out unconsciously if not acted on with conscious intention (Bowlby, 1963). Those bereaved individuals who have tamped any yearning to reclaim proximity to the deceased may find themselves compelled to relate to others as mere substitutes for whom they have lost.

Lucy was not relating to her friends as the individuals they were in and of themselves; she was quietly hoping to place them in her father's stead, effectively rediscovering his personality, and the relationship they had, in others. I seemed to take the bait in our early work together. This enactment of transference and countertransference only colluded with her evasion of the loss-oriented stress of no longer having her father to provide the support she wished were still present. Though we did eventually identify and truncate this pattern, my interest in her career goals was thwarting the necessary process of talking about how *she wanted to still share everything with her father*.

People such as Lucy experience bereavement as a quick transition into restoration-oriented stress. They wish to simply get on with life and shirk the messy, seemingly unproductive emotional elements of mourning. Grief, for them, is devoid of conscious yearning for their loved one's presence. The absence of the deceased is thought of and spoken about as a plain fact: Lucy's father died, period. This approach may look remarkably healthy and adaptive for a while, but it all too often gives way to insidious manifestations of complicated bereavement.

Lucy desperately needed to give herself an occasional break from the stress she was using to distract herself from grief. She was beginning to notice prolonged bouts of exhaustion after overexerting herself at work. In earnest, Lucy was attempting to be independent, to adapt to her father's absence by tackling the demands of her career and of home ownership without her father's support. As she continued to crowd her waking hours with activities rooted in the here and now, I asked her if she ever noticed herself avoiding activities that might bring her father to mind. "Yeah," she said, "it's funny that you ask, 'cause it recently dawned on me that I haven't been to a game at Wrigley Field this year, and I have no plans to go. That's weird for me." Lucy explained that she and her father, both avid Chicago Cubs fans, had an annual tradition of going to at least one baseball game together every season. Being a lifelong Cubs fan myself, I was alarmed. I inquired into the reason for her inhibition. More than anything, she feared that attending a game just as they had always done would bring out memories of the past along with deep feelings of loss she was not ready to sit with. She also expressed guilt about the likelihood that she would cry throughout the game, thus ruining everyone else's time. In a somewhat-defensive response, I joked, "Cubs fans are accustomed to seeing each other cry." (This was in 2015, prior to the Cubs winning the World Series!)

Despite the dread she felt about tapping into her grief, she did not want to be afraid of going back to the Friendly Confines for the rest of her life. Lucy and I soon began designing a personal grief ritual in which she planned to resume going to Wrigley Field like she once did with her father. She planned to use the evening to reflect upon the relationship she lost, but she also decided that it would be meaningful to bring her younger sister to the game with her. As discussed in Chapter 3, if someone is invited to partake in a personal grief ritual, including those that are intended to be emotionally evocative, it is essential that they are a trusted person who will not impede upon the necessity to express feelings.

This type of personal grief ritual facilitates emotional expression about the deceased as the bereaved goes back in time to reminisce about days spent with a loved one. It amounts to a compartmentalized break from the stresses of moving forward with new developments and relationships. Lucy reported that she began to tear up soon after finding her seat in the bleachers, where she and her father preferred to watch the game. As she gazed upon the green grass, Wrigley's iconic scoreboard, and the ivy on the outfield wall which had just started to take on a brown hue as autumn fast approached, Lucy recalled the games she first attended as a child with her father by her side, teaching her how to count balls and strikes. Though she quietly shed tears at a few moments, she thoroughly enjoyed the evening and basked in the opportunity to teach her sister the game she had grown to love. She was relieved to no longer have to fearfully avoid her favorite ballpark . . . and her emotions. Interestingly, it was after this personal grief ritual that she began to consciously protest her father's absence with more fervor and consistency, expressing anger and sadness about how unfair it felt that she lost her biggest fan in life. Some years after we completed our work, I was happy to hear from Lucy again and to learn that she and her sister carried on the tradition of going to Wrigley Field together once every season.

Using symbols to coax out emotional experience and expression

Incorporating symbols into a personal grief ritual opens up facets of emotional experience and expression beyond what verbal communication alone can unveil. Symbolic activities give external form to inner turmoil otherwise felt to be amorphous and indescribable. And interactions with symbolic ties to the past enlist any number of sensory experiences to unearth buried feelings: Music piques the ears with haunting recollections harkening back to days gone by; the familiar tastes and aromas of family recipes awaken bittersweet memories; holding tangible heirlooms or personal possessions once belonging to the dead in one's hands pulls the bereaved to gaze upon and touch remnants of what has been lost.

Mourning customs from nineteenth-century America provide an intimate glimpse into the use of clothing and fabrics as visual symbols of grief. Death was more commonplace in the 1800s than it is today. Infant mortality rates ran rampant, as did death during childbirth, which was the number one cause of female death at that time. Predating wide acceptance of germ theory, a lack of medical sophistication yielded to an abundance of deaths stemming from tuberculosis, influenza, cancer, and pneumonia. Even a simple infected cut could precipitate one's demise! As follows, public acknowledgments of grief were woven into the backdrop of everyday life, often consisting of dark hues that put uncomfortable feelings on display. Members of a community regularly bore witness to these visual representations of loss. The bereaved draped large black linens over the front door and windows of their homes (white cloth was preferred in the event of a child's death). Both men and women shrouded themselves in exclusively black clothing while mourning, often for weeks or months beyond the funeral (Mehaffey, 2006).

The bereaved individual may wish to break from cultural custom and symbolize grief with a color of their choosing that captures what their subjective experience of loss feels like. And besides, there is no worldly consensus regarding which shade of gray best encapsulates grief. Different cultures adorn themselves in clothing of whichever color they believe represents death and mourning. Where Americans and the Japanese use black to symbolize the macabre tones of sorrow, Hindu and Chinese cultures don themselves in white at their funerals, and South Americans generally express grief through green and purple hues.

When helping my clients design personal grief rituals, I often encourage them to include any symbolic objects that represent some meaningful aspect of the relationship they had with the deceased: a picture from an important day, jewelry and watches bequeathed to them, an item used in a shared hobby, food and recipes, clothing, gifts, or family heirlooms passed down from generation to generation. When the aim is to encourage greater emotional expression, it can be helpful to confront what the symbol reminds the bereaved of and explore, in the moment, what emotion it provokes. I have often found that whoever is performing such a ritual will reliably benefit from clasping the symbolic item and staring at it while unpacking whatever emotions it stirs within.

Some symbols cannot be held in one's hands. Music, for instance, proves to be one of the most powerful and evocative representations of a past bond with the deceased that can be woven into many personal grief rituals. Kendrick, a young man in his twenties, came into therapy because he was struggling to access feelings about his friend's sudden death from a car accident. His emotional inhibition was markedly different from the type of indifference Lucy exhibited; Kendrick was petrified by the prospect of feeling his grief. Whether alone or in company with friends and family, he dared not speak a word of the anguish beating in his heart. He reported a recurring nightmare in which, upon realizing that all his teeth were falling out while attending a party, he kept his mouth closed and avoided conversation with friends, tightly holding his loose teeth in place. (Psychoanalysts could have a field day interpreting this dream as a regression to anal fixations and conflicts pertaining to patterns of holding on and letting go. It is not uncommon for grief to register in physical complaints pertaining to muscle systems that alternate between tightening and loosening, such as constipation and irritable bowels. In the case of this dream, one might interpret that the oral cavity is tightening in an effort to hold in what has already been lost.)

I did invite Kendrick to talk about his feelings, but to no surprise, no words came out of his mouth. He did, however, mention that he and his friend Damien shared musical tastes and that he had been shying away from much of the classic rock bands they listened to together. I asked if he would be willing to partition off some time to listen to a song or two that reminded him of Damien. Kendrick agreed and said he would select some music ahead of time that encapsulated the bond they shared. We began the next appointment playing songs by Jimi Hendrix, Grateful Dead, Cream, Fleetwood Mac, and the Band, all of which they discovered together as budding adolescents. Kendrick's eyes teared up as he listened and reminisced about the friend he lost. I was tempted to encourage him to talk about what he was feeling, but I decided to remain quiet. There was no need to wait for him to utter, "I'm sad" or "I miss him." Kendrick genuinely *experienced* his grief for the first time that day, and the prospect of doing so again in the future became more approachable as a result of accessing what music represented about their friendship.

Rituals that limit emotional expression about the deceased

Pop psychology leads some to believe that grief should be given a steady, undeviating outlet lest the mourning process be somehow stifled. Therapeutic interventions may suffer from this misconception at times, as they tend to favor airing out feelings about loss rather than containing them. But sustained venting of painful feelings, if indiscriminately prescribed without considering the individual's specific needs, can pave a path towards a chronic and complicated course of bereavement. The very noises of grief that should be amplified for some – crying, laughter, screaming, using words to pine for the deceased – are better off dampened in others.

Death rites and funerals around the world are structured in a manner that allows a circumscribed period of time for expressing grief, followed by efforts to curb any further outpouring of distress about the loss. Indeed, culture regularly dictates how long formal mourning should last and when, precisely, it should cease. Specific timelines vary greatly; Taoists typically mourn for a period of forty-nine days, whereas Muslims may only do so for three. These customs draw mourning behaviors to a decisive close and subsequently encourage a resumption of joyful living.

The bereaved individual may wish to deploy a similar approach to contain emotional expression within the personal grief rituals they design. Feelings about loss can be approached within whatever measure of time the individual chooses, be it a particular hour of the day, a span of ten minutes reserved for activities and symbols that reliably evoke sorrow, or a meaningful date on the calendar. And the bereaved can return to these delimited moments as needed. Holidays, birthdays, and other meaningful dates can encompass grief within a boundary of twenty-four hours every year if desired. Like a funeral that begins and ends at fixed times, a day reserved for mourning invites grief that is to be felt today without bleeding into tomorrow.

Special life events are particularly well-suited for this type of time-limited evocation. However, it may be preferrable to only reserve *part* of a special day for difficult feelings so as to safeguard celebrations and festivities from being engulfed in pain. The bereaved has good reason to be concerned about a shadow of sullen gloom hanging over a wedding, a graduation ceremony, a vacation, or a holiday family gathering. Rather than willing oneself to not acknowledge emotions at all, a strategy that is almost guaranteed to backfire, I often encourage my patients to initiate simple rituals that put aside a small amount of time in a specific location to recognize what they are genuinely feeling during a meaningful occasion.

Rene lost both of her parents a year prior to getting married. While preparing for her wedding, she worried that their absence would tug at her heartstrings and leave her white-knuckling her way through the day in hopes of not bursting into tears at an inopportune moment. She and her fiancé planned to arrange framed pictures of her parents on a separate table where others could pause and reflect upon their passing. Amid the day's tight schedule, they reserved fifteen minutes after the ceremony to look at the old photos of her mother and father. Rene let herself cry and lean upon her husband's shoulder for a brief moment. Having put aside time for this emotional outlet, Rene was able to enjoy dining with her family and dancing with her friends without having to pretend that she wasn't heartbroken about her parents not being able to see their daughter getting married.

Anniversary reactions: When to evoke and when to limit emotional expression

The sight of winter's first falling snow rekindles old memories of building snowmen and gathering with family for the holidays. Fireworks erupt overhead, and the smell of smoke transports us back to summer evenings spent marveling at the illuminated night sky. The cadence of seasons, with their re-emerging traditions and familiar symbols, awakens a bittersweet mixture of nostalgia and grief for what has come and passed. Psychoanalytic writers have long reflected upon the phenomenon of anniversary reactions in relation to mourning and how mere dates on a calendar can trigger the recall of repressed feelings about lost relationships that otherwise remain locked away in annals of the past (Hull et al., 1993; Pollock, 1970).

Dates redolent with sorrowful reflections should be approached with caution. For those bereaved individuals who err towards excessive loss-oriented stress, anniversaries unearth affect-laden memories whose intensity may threaten to overwhelm them with further pining for the past. In such instances, anniversaries should perhaps be treated less as times to reminisce and more as markers in time that the bereaved strive to move beyond with new activities grounded in the present (see Chapter 7). But for the majority of the bereaved, including those consumed by a disproportionate amount of restoration-oriented stress, anniversaries and other meaningful moments throughout the year provide opportunities to give pause and feel grief about the deceased's absence.

Matthew, a man in his early forties, came to therapy three months after his sister succumbed to chronic bronchitis between Thanksgiving and Christmas. The first year following her death was notably difficult for him, although his wife, friends, and family would have never suspected. Matthew pushed through one holiday and meaningful date after another, dodging his emotions at every turn. He kept himself busy taking care of his two young children and tending to his career. But as Thanksgiving loomed nearer, approximately a year after his sister's death, he suspected it was high time to finally confront the grief he had been hiding from. Family gatherings had become reliably tense affairs during which he exerted enormous energy glossing over his feelings with platitudes and small talk about trivial events in sports and the news. Nonetheless, these efforts to sidestep his overwhelming sense of loss had only grown more unbearable and unavoidable. And with Thanksgiving being the holiday that he and his sister bonded over the most, Matthew had good reason to suspect that grief would inevitably burst forth in chaotic fashion if not given proper release.

Matthew and I discussed how he could put aside time early in the morning of Thanksgiving to visit the mausoleum where his sister was buried and let his guard down, free from the burdens of the workplace and his concerns that a great show of emotion would spoil the holidays for his family. He also planned to say a simple toast before the meal to acknowledge the first year of his sister's absence at the table. Matthew benefited immensely from approaching his feelings during the anniversary. He learned to better trust that he could handle his grief when it emerges, especially during evocative occasions. Personal grief rituals such as these not only provide catharsis but also instill the bereaved with confidence and the simple knowledge that small amounts of time can be used to compartmentalize otherwise large feelings of loss and sorrow.

Attending to specific emotions: Anger

A wide array of emotions must be expressed and experienced in order to properly process the full breadth of mourning. Individuals like Lucy and Kendrick and Matthew benefit from reactivating their *entire* emotional repertoire and channeling sundry feelings through evocative activities and meaningful symbols. In other instances, the impediment to healthy mourning lies only in a specific emotion that has been tamped down, be it sorrow, anger, fear, or joy. Personal grief rituals can be most effectively tailored to what is hindering the individual if we understand which emotions are coming forth easily and which are being held back. Anger certainly deserves special consideration, as it is particularly susceptible to inhibitions stemming from both societal mores and personal conflicts residing within the individual.

Culture plays a key role in giving voice to certain feelings in mourning while muzzling others. Anger has proven to be one such target for censure. The adage "Don't speak ill of the dead" spans epochs of human history and has been incorporated into many peoples' values and beliefs. Often attributed to the Greek philosopher Chilon of Sparta, circa 600 BCE, *de mortuis mil nisi bonum* is translated as "Of the dead, nothing unless good." This prohibition is, for many, rooted in fears of the deceased's lingering spirit and its proclivity for malevolence. Amid the strain of grief, anxious concerns about the dead using supernatural powers to retaliate against the living run wild. The living are implored to not goad the dead's wrath with reproaches. Thus, many bereaved individuals remain reticent to utter any mention of anger, frustration, or disappointment towards those they have lost.

Jewish culture prohibits expressions of anger because the dead can no longer defend themselves against an onslaught of criticisms and attacks, and so it becomes the responsibility of the living to defend their honor. Native Americans consider any mention of the dead's name to be a disturbance of the spirit. Christians are prohibited from speaking ill of the dead because such remarks are considered hypocritical, judgmental, and devoid of God's grace. In the book of Titus, it states:

> For we ourselves were once foolish, disobedient, led astray, slaves to various passions and pleasures, passing our days in malice and envy, hated by others and hating one another. But when the goodness and loving kindness of God our Savior appeared, he saved us, not because of works done by us in righteousness, but according to his own mercy.
>
> (King James Bible, 2008, Titus, 3:3)

Though it may be unpleasant to voice anger, resentment, disappointments, or frustrations about the deceased, it is necessary to give these negatively tinged emotions their due discharge if the feeling is naturally there. Persistent and unchanging anger, many argue, is one of the hallmarks of complicated bereavement (Shear & Mulhare, 2008; Simon, 2012). Left unexpressed, it festers and becomes increasingly inimical to the mourning process. It is bound to find an alternate route towards expression if need be, even if leveled at an undeserving bystander. One's ire may be directed towards surviving family members, friends, coworkers and colleagues, various physicians, even a stranger standing in line to get a cup of coffee. But the result is reliably unsatisfying. A scattershot of anger at the living fails to hit its true target.

In a seminal work titled *Mourning and Melancholia*, Sigmund Freud (1917) observed that the naturally self-restorative processes of mourning can careen into a melancholic state if anger regarding the deceased is misdirected towards oneself. Melancholia, referred to today as a major depressive disorder, is indeed characterized by internal attributions of emptiness, worthlessness, and moral inferiority. But how is it that the bereaved comes to hold oneself in such low regard while attempting to mourn a loss?

Freud posited that unconscious ambivalence towards the deceased is the culprit that derails mourning's intended course. Alongside feelings of love towards the departed attachment figure, equally strong feelings of hate murmur beneath the surface. But if one is uneasy about consciously acknowledging these mixed feelings, reproach is turned inward towards the self in an act of defensive displacement. The bereaved regard themselves in light of what they actually feel about the deceased, effectively identifying with the dead. And so Freud famously quipped, "Thus, the shadow of the object fell upon the ego" (p. 249). It may seem like Sigmund was merely waxing poetic, but research eight decades later substantiated his claims: Intrusive thoughts and obsessive preoccupations are at their highest levels with bereaved individuals who had a highly conflicted attachment with the deceased (Worden, 1996).

Whether anger is held back because of external pressures or internal conflicts, personal grief rituals can draw out one's ire in earnest. It is imperative that these practices amount to more than unbridled fits of rage. They are not intended to be a wholesale condemnation of the deceased's character or to imply that the relationship was devoid of genuine warmth. Instead, activities and symbols used in such rituals can help coax out a healthy balance of mixed feelings – love, sorrow, frustration, disappointment . . . and anger – tied to a multifaceted relationship. Love and hate need not be a zero-sum game.

One approach to this type of personal grief ritual centers on conveying anger *to* the deceased through illusory conversation. This can certainly be facilitated within a therapy session, but the bereaved may wish to do so in a meaningful location in private. Jennifer, a woman in her late fifties, had lost her son to lung cancer that metastasized to his brain and bones. Kameron was only thirty-six years old. He smoked heavily from the time he was an adolescent, and it was suspected that this precocious use of tobacco was largely responsible for his early demise. Jennifer experienced a tense Christmas dinner with her family soon after her son's death. The evening was filled with awkward attempts to avoid any uncomfortable feelings about Kameron's absence at the dining room table. While Jennifer was cleaning up at the end of the night, her surviving son shared his concern that she was struggling to acknowledge her grief. He urged her to seek out professional help, and Jennifer began therapy with me shortly after the new year.

A short and cheerfully upbeat woman, Jennifer always entered my office with a smile on her face. She seemed to bounce up and down while sitting on the couch. Like clockwork, she began every appointment by pulling out a list of things to talk about: "I'm wondering if it makes sense to stay in the city now that Kameron isn't here?" "How can I devote more time to my other son?" "When people ask me if I have children, should I say one or two?"

Jennifer's attempts to cope with loss perfectly demonstrate what an excess of *restoration-oriented stress* looks like. She seldom addressed feelings of grief; at most, she would allude to a vague sense of sadness. I would then ask her to express more, but she would invariably pivot back to further explorations of how she would navigate the remainder of her life. Merely asking Jennifer to talk about feelings was leading her nowhere.

During one appointment, Jennifer was moving through her usual list of goals and questions about the future when she suddenly detoured and said, "I sometimes just get really frustrated about the smoking. I gave him a hard time about it once or twice, but he just wouldn't listen. He wouldn't take it seriously." Jennifer was clearly irritated. I asked her to expand on what she was feeling, but to little surprise, she drew a blank and added, "There's something there, but . . . I don't know." I had watched this play out often in our work together: Jennifer would begin exploring uncomfortable feelings and then quickly revert back to her peppy presentation. Before she could steer the conversation away from her upset, I simply observed that she seemed angry at Kameron. "Well," she said, "I do wish I could tell him. The feeling is there, but you can't exactly talk with family over the holidays about how angry you are at your dead son." I invited Jennifer to consider putting aside time in an upcoming session to have an imaginary conversation with her son and to let herself express all that she had been harboring since his passing, including feelings of anger. She took to the idea with enthusiasm but was understandably confused about how to get started. She asked, "Should I talk to you like you are Kameron? Should I close my eyes?" I responded by pointing to the empty chair against the wall in my office.

Empty chair technique is a therapeutic intervention used in gestalt therapy to help clients work through interpersonal conflicts involving others who are not physically present. The client is encouraged to communicate in the direction of the empty chair *as if* the relevant party is actually sitting there ready to listen. It can be used to practice initiating a conversation, to release bottled-up emotions towards someone from one's past, or even to speak to oneself from a more compassionate perspective. Grief counselors have long relied upon empty chair technique to help bereaved clients talk honestly *with* the deceased about the many thoughts and feelings they cannot share with anyone else, and this method has been shown to be notably helpful in clinical settings (Field & Horowitz, 1998; Ochsner, 2016). I have come to trust that this therapeutic intervention can be a beneficial and meaningful component of a personal grief ritual.

Jennifer was quite eager to unload the anger she had been carrying since Kameron had fallen ill. I watched her rock back and forth in agitation as she stared at the empty chair in my office, uncertain as to what she wanted to say. Her fury was palpable. Jennifer patiently searched for words to convey to her son how much she missed him and how upset she was about the choices he made that ultimately robbed her of his company. Statements such as "I wish you didn't smoke so much" and "You should have listened to me" spewed forth like so much bile. As she continued her imaginary conversation with Kameron, she squeaked out a few angry admissions of embarrassment about having to repeatedly tell friends and coworkers that her son died because he began smoking at such a young age. Lastly, Jennifer peppered in expressions of love for her son and compassion for an addiction that seemed to be beyond his control.

Jennifer only partook in this activity once in therapy with me. After we reflected upon how helpful it had been, she decided to create an ongoing personal grief ritual that she could carry out by herself as needed. She settled upon holding an imaginary conversation with Kameron prior to family gatherings where his absence would likely stoke cross feelings. She and I soon discovered that the anger she had been holding on to was expending itself rather quickly. The heat of her frustrations had not, in fact, engulfed her in flames. Successive conversations with Kameron yielded an ever-dwindling intensity of anger towards her son's undoing and gave way to the persistent love she felt for her boy. By the time Christmas rolled around again, she no longer felt the need to exorcise these demons, nor did she feel the need to come into therapy with a list of questions about how to move on. She already had.

Verbal expressions of anger may suffice for some, but the bereaved may prefer turning to nonverbal outlets for a deeper, more visceral embodiment of their displeasure. It is often helpful to direct such fiery emotions towards meaningful symbols. Inanimate objects representing that which is irksome can be relinquished or even destroyed. That which contributed mightily to the deceased's poor health and ultimate death, such as junk food or a half-full pack of cigarettes, can be aggressively disposed of into a trash bin. Items reminiscent of bad memories can be ripped apart, stepped on, or shattered onto the concrete. Remnants of some frustrating aspect of the relationship can be buried beneath the ground or burned into a swirl of ashes. Many of my bereaved patients over the years have used photos, items of clothing, or notes from the deceased to write down the specific reason for their anger with the deceased before setting the object ablaze and basking in its flames. On many occasions, they have gleefully taken videos of the event and brought them in to therapy appointments to show me.

Volkan's notion of *linking objects* elucidates why relinquishing or destroying certain items can provide a cleansing purge of raw anger. Throughout the course of mourning, many free-floating emotions will arise that the bereaved wishes to tamp down. He may attempt to repress and deny critical thoughts and feelings towards the dead. He may even direct anger at an undeserving person who can absorb the attack, including one's own self. The bereaved may also establish distance from unsavory feelings by injecting them into inanimate objects external to himself that symbolically encapsulate what he wishes to no longer harbor within. These linking objects are then monitored like the original untrustworthy feeling that was threatening to burst forth and wreak havoc. It is a doomed strategy. Persistent efforts to exert control over anger only leave these feelings unresolved, lingering in wait to manifest at inopportune times.

Carina, who was discussed in the previous chapter, tended to punish herself with sharp rebukes for having failed to safeguard her husband, Leonard, from illness and death. This was completely baseless, of course. She had done everything within her power to care for him throughout his battle with leukemia. It begged the question: Who was the true object of her fury?

Carina and I had already decided it was important for her to discard any superfluous belongings that were cluttering her home before she moved out. Among other things she brought into my office to get rid of, there were boxes filled with medical supplies – ointments, pamphlets, pills, gauzes, and various physical therapy devices to help him counter symptoms of neuropathy – that Leonard had taken home from the hospital. As Carina began throwing these items into a trash can, a torrent of obscenities about Leonard's team of doctors poured out of her mouth. This gentle and kind elderly woman was releasing wave after wave of frustration and resentment about the hopeful prognosis the doctors had offered, the painful procedures Leonard endured, and the cold tone with which they eventually told her that there was nothing more they could do for him. She also let forth a cascade of anger towards Leonard for the simple fact that he died and left her alone, a common expression of protest in mourning. When Carina was done throwing away the last item, she looked up at me with a self-conscious look of embarrassment and said, "I can't believe I just said all those horrible things."

Insofar as linking objects retain ambivalence, efforts must be made to *extract* mixed feelings of love alongside unconscious anger towards the deceased. Personal grief rituals can facilitate so much more than the discharge of unpalatable words about all that is felt. They can also be designed around the performance of charged activities to embody what has been kept quiet. The ritual relinquishes and establishes distance from the concrete object itself as well as the affect it encases.

Some will reach deep into their psyches only to find that there is no ambivalent mixture of positive and negative feelings waiting to be excavated. It may very well be that an unhealthy relationship has left them with nothing more than seething hatred and a desire to wrest themselves free of old attachments. In such cases, the individual should look to develop personal grief rituals that emphasize leaving the relationship behind them as they move forward (see Chapter 7). They may even opt to use acts of destruction to aggressively renounce those aspects of the relationship too unpalatable to express with words.

Most will find that as they sift through the innumerable feelings that color their grief, like so many granules of sand that seem indistinguishable from one another, an assortment of contrasting emotions begin to emerge. Tender pangs of sorrow and pining for reunion are intermingled with rougher feelings of resentment, disappointment, frustration, and anger. And if the bereaved continues to comb through the grains of emotion they hold in their shaky hand, they may soon find themselves gazing upon particles of relief, excitement, happiness, and joy that slowly come into focus.

Attending to specific emotions: Joy

Traditional jazz funerals of New Orleans and Cajun culture are characterized by the unique accompaniment of a brass band that plays somber music as the procession leads the bereaved from church to the cemetery (Sakakeeny, 2010). The music's slow tempo and minor key coincide with the melancholy timbre of each mourner's cries as loved ones are bid farewell. Shortly after the body is buried, saxophones, tubas, trumpets, and trombones launch into more uplifting jazz standards. The very sound of mourning shifts from a sorrowful tone to one of jubilation! A celebratory atmosphere permeates what remains of the day as attendees dance and exude joy while walking away from the burial site, sometimes culminating in a party held in the deceased's honor. This sequence of behaviors symbolizes movement away from grief and towards the happiness that life will continue to offer. In *The Music of Black Americans* (Southern, 1996), Eileen Southern wrote:

> On the way to the cemetery it was customary to play very slowly and mournfully a dirge, or an "old Negro spiritual" such as "Nearer My God to Thee," but on the return from the cemetery, the band would strike up a rousing, "When the Saints Go Marching In," or a ragtime song such as "Didn't He Ramble." The renowned New Orleans jazz musician Sidney Bechet stated, after observing the celebrations of the jazz funeral, "Music here is as much a part of death as it is of life."
>
> (p. 341)

Traditionally, grief rituals of the Zulu people of postapartheid South Africa have been solemn and quiet affairs. Mourners return from the funeral and partake in a cleansing ritual in which they wash off dust from the burial before re-entering the home. But mourning is by no means behind them. Anywhere from one week to three months is devoted to nothing but persistent grief. However long this formal phase of mourning is to last, normal life is abruptly frozen in place. The bereaved are to abandon many of their day-to-day behaviors during this time. All household items that give off a reflection such as television sets and mirrors are covered. Social activity is limited to bare essentials. The bereaved are not even permitted to speak or make noise until mourning is officially declared complete (Kotze et al., 2012).

Meanwhile, a younger generation of South Africans has developed a vastly different kind of mourning ritual that, akin to the New Orleans jazz funeral, encourages a joyful emotional experience alongside the more sullen and gloomy expressions of grief. Referred to as an *after-tears party*, family and friends of the deceased gather after the funeral to remember the dead and celebrate their life with food, music, alcohol, and dancing (Abruzzini, 2017). The mood is unmistakably light in contrast to the heavy burden of sorrow.

This newer practice has given rise to no shortage of controversy and disapproval, particularly among older generations, who see such raucous behavior disrespectful to the dead and as being antithetical to traditional African values about mourning. But it is easy to understand how a younger generation can experience the austere practices of old as unduly restrictive and stale. For instance, children and those who are not married are usually barred from attending funerals in South Africa. And for widows who have lost a husband, tradition has required them to mourn for an entire year, effectively imposing oppressive strictures. These emotional and behavioral restrictions have rightly given rise to the creation of a unique ritual that meets the needs of individuals who wish to mourn in a more lively atmosphere.

One of the most common misunderstandings about mourning is that its emotional landscape is a barren wasteland of dread and despondent gloom. Sadness, anger, and anxiety are considered inevitable stages to be worked through. Positive emotions seem to only await at the end of the journey and often consist of nothing more than the flat state of acceptance, a defeated soul who has finally resigned to reality. This is an unfortunate oversight, as emotions with a positive tinge play their own crucial role in the mourning process. The sheer absence of the deceased naturally evokes pain for many. But absence may also evoke a great sense of *relief* upon no longer having to observe a loved one in pain, *excitement* about being able to spend less time in the hospital and more time on life-fulfilling hobbies and relationships, or *joy* in reflecting on a cherished relationship. And for those who managed a highly conflictual or abusive relationship with the now-departed, absence may usher in a great sense of *liberation*.

Varied and seemingly contradictory feelings actually work in concert with and give way to one another. Happiness can be derived from the nostalgia of fond memories and an appreciation for having had such a meaningful relationship, which then yields upset about no longer being able to accrue good times. Immense sadness need not overshadow joy. The buoyancy of relief and excitement does not lift the entire burden of emptiness, yet the bereaved may struggle to acknowledge these mixed feelings. Manifestations of emotions with a positive valence create a great deal of conflict for those who keep the true range of their grief hidden behind a thin veil of negative, socially approved anguish.

Why is it that some bereaved individuals evade happiness or bite their tongues before broadcasting ongoing enthusiasm for life after a loss? Often, this is quite simply the product of social pressures to act the part of the downtrodden and bereft that others expect to see. Harking back to earlier examples of cultures whose rituals demand an outward show of distress, one cannot help but wonder about how often genuinely positive emotions within the individual are quashed in an effort to establish social cohesion with fellow mourners. Internal pressures may be to blame in other instances, as the bereaved can come to feel guilty about spontaneous behaviors that reveal happiness despite having lost a loved one. Many of my bereaved patients have addressed their concerns about letting people see any indication that they are doing reasonably well, as they worry this might suggest that the loss apparently meant nothing to them. Positive emotions, they fear, are tantamount to a betrayal of the deceased. In such instances, negative emotional expression can amount to an inauthentic and compulsory show of undying devotion to the dead.

Stringent avoidance of positive emotion over time has a pernicious effect on mourning. An unwillingness to let in feelings of happiness or excitement contributes to a chronic pattern in which the bereaved believes they are obliged to remain unwavering in their misery. Personal grief rituals can counter this impediment by pushing the bereaved to re-engage in joyful activity that reasserts one's zest for life. It may prove beneficial to fold into the ritual others who can bear witness to the individual's capacity for joy that exists alongside the ongoing pangs of grief.

Tameeka, a hardworking woman in her thirties, sought out therapy after losing her mother to gallbladder cancer. She was at her mother's side during all three years of her ordeal and nursed her at home in the last weeks of her life. Tameeka contacted with me through email shortly after, saying that she had been struggling to deal with her grief: "I can't really talk about it." Her mother had always been a beacon of wisdom and guidance, particularly when it came to Tameeka's promising career. She felt lost and misguided without her. Soon after we began our work together, an outpouring of sadness and despair ensued, but she still felt that some aspect of her grief remained unaddressed – an itch left unscratched.

After a couple of months of therapy, Tameeka reported an incident that she found curious. She had recently gone shopping for an outfit to wear to an upcoming gala party for work. Upon returning home, she hung up the dress she bought, took a step back to look at it, and felt mystified as to what she had purchased. "I got a *mauve* dress! A *mauve* dress?" Tameeka paused in anticipation of a validating response from me. I only stared back at her blankly. Seeing as how the nuances of neither colors nor fashion are my strong suit, I asked her to clarify what mauve is. "It's kind of a dull color. It's like purple, but more gray and . . . blah." She added, "That's not the kind of color I usually wear to these things." Her eyes welled up with tears. "That's not how my mother taught me to dress."

Tameeka elaborated on how her mother had always encouraged her to choose outfits for professional events that were bright and bold and celebratory. But here was this *mauve* dress staring her down. I asked, "Why do you think you bought a dress in that color?" Without hesitation, she responded, "Because of the cameras." Tameeka explained that there was going to be a bevy of celebrities at this event and that the evening news would likely send reporters to cover it. She fretted about the possibility that people she knew would see her having fun on television. And what's worse, they'd see her wearing a bright outfit! I offered my best attempt at empathizing with her conflict: "The mauve dress would ensure that you look like you are mourning, that you haven't returned to your usually vibrant wardrobe. You feel pressured to look like you are unhappy."

Tameeka's befuddling choice of attire was beginning to make sense to her. She still grieved her mother's absence, but she genuinely wanted to resume enjoying her life. Plus, the memory of her mother's advice about how to celebrate and dress with confidence filled her with warmth. Positive emotions persisted in spite of loss and reminded her of everything from her relationship with her mother that she would forever be able to hold in mind. We agreed that the gala event needed to be a meaningful expression of where she was in the mourning process. It would be an unabashed display of genuine happiness despite her pain. Tameeka soon exchanged the mauve dress for one that was, as she described it, "bright purple." Familiar with that color, I smiled and nodded in recognition.

Tameeka's plan to exhibit happiness amid mourning demonstrates how some personal grief rituals can be designed to showcase an aspect of the lost relationship that has left a positive impression upon the bereaved. She ultimately wore a bright dress to memorialize the self-confidence her mother imparted her way. This ritual was all the more important in that she allowed herself to enjoy life in a public setting, countering her fear that only negative emotion could be displayed for others to see.

There is one last type of personal grief ritual to consider: Those that help to reclaim fond memories and experience the positive emotions they awaken. It is profound to observe just how often bereaved individuals seem to repress positive memories of the time they spent with loved attachment figures who are now gone. Recollections of good times are an essential component of a healthy mourning process, a counterbalance of bittersweet remembrances and funny stories to offset the heavy pain of loss. Even as these reflections upon the past may bring a smile to one's face, they are often defended against because of a painful yearning for more good times.

Personal grief rituals can be creatively designed to venture back into the past and recapture warm memories otherwise relegated to a distant and forgotten past. One approach is to use meaningful symbols and representations of the now-foregone relationship. The bereaved may portion off time to look through pictures and photo albums of time spent with the deceased or gather with others and regale one another with stories.

A variation on this type of ritual involves re-enacting activities once done with the deceased so as to stir up muscle memory and remind oneself of the relationship they once enjoyed. The bereaved is often surprised to find that these activities do more than dredge up pleasant feelings connected to the past. They may imbue the actor with a subjective sense of *presence*, an illusory experience of ongoing interaction with the deceased that functions in tandem with positive feelings of comfort, nostalgia, or a sense of being moved.

Perhaps Lucy's visit to Wrigley Field allowed her to suspend disbelief for a moment and find solace in the sense that her father was once again watching a baseball game at her side. In the next chapter, we will revisit Tameeka's journey through mourning as she strove to revive the tender feelings of attachment to her mother by going shopping "with [her] mom." Matthew, too, will show us how he took part in his sister's hobbies after her death so as to "keep her alive" and buoy his spirits through the holidays.

Each bereaved individual must sort out and cope with the kaleidoscopic array of emotions that color their grief and emerge upon confronting absence. Now living in a world more empty than before, they search for loved ones in the external environment to no avail. They cry out in anger and sadness for a bond they can no longer lean upon. They may even resonate with an odd sense of happiness in letting go of the loving ties they were grateful to have. But each individual may also benefit from discovering, in their own meaningful way, that a piece of the relationship they lost still resides within.

References

Abruzzini, M. (2017, January 4). The Evolution of after-tears parties in South Africa. *SevenPonds*. https://blog.sevenponds.com/cultural-perspectives/the-evolution-of-after-tears-parties-in-south-africa

Boelen, P. A., & Klugkist, I. (2011). Cognitive behavioral variables mediate the associations of neuroticism and attachment insecurity with prolonged grief disorder severity. *Anxiety, Stress, and Coping*, *24*, 291–307.

Bowlby, J. (1963). Pathological mourning and childhood mourning. *Journal of the American Psychoanalytic Association*, *11*, 500–541.

Field, N. P., & Horowitz, M. J. (1998). Applying an empty-chair monologue paradigm to examine unresolved grief. *Psychiatry: Interpersonal and Biological Processes*, *61*(4), 279–287.

Freud, S. (1917). Mourning and melancholia. *Standard Edition*, *14*, 243–258. Hogarth Press.

Hitchens, C., Mann, W., & Amis, M. (2011). *The quotable Hitchens: From alcohol to Zionism: The very best of Christopher Hitchens*. Da Capo Press.

Hull, J. W., Lane, R. C., & Gibbons, B. (1993). Early object loss and "secret anniversaries of the heart." *Psychoanalytic Psychology*, *10*(1), 77–91.

Kerrigan, M. (2017). *The history of death*. Amber Books.

King James Bible. (2008). Oxford University Press. (Original work published 1769).

Kotze, E., Els, L., & Rajuili-Masilo, N. (2012). "Women . . . mourn and men carry on": African women storying mourning practices: A South African example. *Death Studies*, *36*, 742–766.

Kunkel, A. D., & Dennis, M. R. (2003). Grief consolation in eulogy rhetoric: An integrative framework. *Death Studies*, *27*, 1–38.

Lee, H. S. (1996). Change in funeral customs in contemporary Korea. *Korea Journal*, *36*(2), 49–60.

Mehaffey, K. R. (2006). *Rachel weeping: Mourning in nineteenth century America*. Moss Rose Books, LLC.

Ochsner, J. K. (2016). Meditations on the empty chair: The form of mourning and reverie. *American Imago*, *73*(2), 131–163.

O'Connor, M. F., Wellisch, D. K., Stanton, A. L., Eisenberger, N. I., Irwin, M. R., & Lieberman, M. D. (2008). Craving love? Enduring grief activates brain's reward center. *NeuroImage*, *42*(2), 969–972.

Pollock, G. H. (1970). Anniversary reactions, trauma, and mourning. *Psychoanalytic Quarterly*, *39*(3), 347–371.

Rosenblatt, P. C. (1997). Grief in small-scale societies. In P. Laungani & W. Young (Eds.), *Death and bereavement across cultures* (pp. 27–51). Routledge.

Sakakeeny, M. (2010). Under the bridge: An orientation to soundscapes in New Orleans. *Ethnomusicology*, *54*(1), 1–27.

Schenck, L. K., Eberle, K. M., & Rings, J. A. (2016). Insecure attachment styles and complicated grief severity: Applying what we know to inform future directions. *OMEGA – Journal of Death and Dying, 73*(3), 231–249.
Shear, M. K., & Mulhare, E. (2008). Complicated grief. *Psychiatric Annals, 38*, 662–670.
Simon, N. M. (2012). Is complicated grief a post-loss stress disorder? *Depression and Anxiety, 29*, 541–544.
Southern, E. (1996). *The music of black Americans: A history* (3rd ed.). W. W. Norton & Company.
Stroebe, M., & Schut, H. (1999). The dual process model of coping with bereavement: Rationale and description. *Death Studies, 23*, 197–224.
Stroebe, M., Schut, H., & Stroebe, W. (2005). Attachment in coping with bereavement: A theoretical integration. *Review of General Psychology, 9*, 48–66.
Wellenkamp, J. C. (1991). Fallen leaves: Death and grieving in Toraja. In D. R. Counts & D. A. Counts (Eds.), *Coping with the final tragedy: Cultural variation in dying and grieving* (pp. 113–134). Baywood Publishing Company.
Worden, J. W. (1996). *Children and grief: When a parent dies*. Guilford Press.
Worden, J. W. (2008). *Grief counseling and grief therapy: A handbook for the mental health practitioner* (4th ed.). Springer Publishing Company.

Chapter 6

Continuing bonds

Rituals that create an enduring connection

Vince was only forty-one years old when his wife of the same age, Sophie, died suddenly from a ruptured brain aneurysm. The morning of her death had begun as inconspicuously as any other Saturday. Vince and Sophie sat together at their small kitchen table and took their time finishing breakfast. They clutched cups of coffee, stared out the window, and discussed their plans to enjoy the crisp fall weather with a long stroll through a nearby nature preserve. Vince recalled how nonchalant Sophie was as she slowly put her coffee down, closed her eyes, and asked to be taken to the hospital because of a gnawing headache that abruptly ceased her calm. Sophie was pronounced dead within an hour.

Vince soon faced a barrage of blunt confrontations with reality. He managed all announcements of her death, the funeral arrangements and religious rites, a separate secular memorial service, Sophie's estate, and plans for her cremation. While on bereavement leave from work, he sat alone at the small kitchen table for hours each morning and read from the ever-mounting pile of condolence cards. He whittled away the afternoons fielding drawn-out phone calls from sympathetic friends and family. With little else to occupy his mind, the spaces between these activities left him besieged by uncontrollable fits of crying. He ate small meals throughout the day. He lay awake at night. Vince was engulfed in the pains of no longer having Sophie by his side.

But Vince's suffering began to lift. Daily acknowledgments of loss helped move him through the most acute phases of shock. The intensity of his grief expended itself and erupted less frequently. As his appetite returned, and as sleep crept back into his nights, he decided to go back to work, his singular respite from the ache of loneliness he felt while sitting at home. The hours between shifts were a dreadful vacuum. When I asked Vince how he felt he was doing, he only shrugged his shoulders and uttered, "I feel empty." He could talk with ease about how he missed Sophie's physical presence, her touch, the timbre of her voice, her scent, but he yearned for something he could not put his finger on.

Some eleven years prior to her passing, Vince and Sophie had met on the job and quickly became inseparable. Their desks adjoined, they sat next to

DOI: 10.4324/9781351204873-6

each other every day. She had always left a canary-yellow sweater draped over her chair in case she got cold, and upon returning to work, Vince found that his colleagues had not removed the sweater she left there on what proved to be her final day. Vince was not at all unsettled by the sight of Sophie's sweater. In fact, he was happy to see it waiting for him and decided to leave it hanging off her old chair for weeks after coming back. He commented on how the comfort he derived from furtive glances at the sweater got him through the workday. I asked him to share his thoughts about why this gave him such ease and what it meant to him to see her sweater there as it had always been. A curious grin stretched across his face as he shrugged his shoulders and said, "I don't know."

Rapprochement in mourning: The absence-and-presence dialectic

Mourning often entails a paradoxical process of accepting a loved one's absence and maintaining a sense of their presence, of letting go while holding on. Even as the bereaved manages to separate from the past and grasp what lies ahead, he reaches back in time to tether himself to some semblance of what has been left behind. A father's guidance continues to reverberate in the ears. The company of a dear friend is still felt to be at one's side. The bereaved stares reality in the face, with its cold and unforgiving glare, and, in a defiant show of protest, continues to nurture an illusory connection to the dead. The hallucination is held in delicate balance with full awareness of the horrible truth.

Denial lingers because the reality of absence cannot be endured for long if laid bare. Days following the deceased's passing accumulate and weigh ever heavier on the mind; the further one gets from the last moment of contact, the deeper the pangs of separation grow. This passing of time creates a subjective experience of intolerable distance, like a toddler who revolts against being apart from her mother for too long. The bereaved feel as if they are careening further away into a silent abyss where they can no longer hear the deceased's voice; old ties fade into a quiet decrescendo. And so a rapprochement crisis ensues after loss, complete with its telltale conflict between the drive to venture away and, upon doing so, subsequent fears of separation from the past. It is then imperative to collapse this distance between the past and present with a compromise. Any shows of protest that sought to reclaim the deceased's *actual* presence of old must bend to reality, but the attachment schema can be revised to search instead for *a symbolic representation of the deceased's presence*.

Mourning certainly demands that one come to terms with the sobering truth of permanent loss. Fantasies of ongoing access to attachment figures exactly as they always were, nestled deep in dark waters, must be brought into contact with sunlight. But if there is to be robust adaptation to loss, objective reality alone proves to be flat and vapid. Merely acknowledging absence – here yesterday, gone today – with no subjective sense of presence is a bloodless capitulation to death, a whimper of defeat devoid of any vigor. Continuing bonds imbue life back into the fight. A revival of past interactions with an attachment figure emboldens the individual to move forward with strength. William Worden (2008) has gone so far as to say that, alongside the importance of accepting the reality of loss (Task I), maintaining an enduring connection with the deceased (Task IV) represents an equally crucial task of mourning. The blurry balancing act of *absence-and-presence* colors the experience of a healthy life after loss.

Still, there will always be great tension between acceptance and protest. If the bereaved embraces the felt presence of continuing bonds, she wonders, must she forfeit her grip on reality? If she holds tight to the truth of absence, will she have to let go of the deceased forever? Numerous cultures' customs and grief rituals reconcile this tension by granting absence and presence equal footing in mourning. Acts of ongoing connection to the deceased are firmly couched in acknowledgment that the deceased is no longer there in the form they once assumed.

Some cultural rituals ensure that the bereaved literally stay close to the deceased's remains. The people of Apayao, a northern province of the Philippines, bury their dead beneath the kitchens in their homes (Vanoverbergh, 1939). In Kiribati, a small island country in the Pacific Ocean, bereaved family members lay out the deceased's body in the home for a minimum of three days before burial; then, several months after interment in the ground, the corpse is exhumed so that the skull can be detached from the body, treated with oils, polished, and displayed upon a shelf in the home, where it will stay indefinitely. Family members regularly carry on conversations with the skull and make offerings of food or tobacco for the deceased's spirit to enjoy. A surviving child or spouse may even continue to sleep near the skeletal remains or carry the skull with them during important occasions (Talu, 1998).

As discussed in previous chapters, many cultures observe a prolonged liminal period of time between biological death and eventual acknowledgment of death's true arrival. This interim, which may span a stretch of months or even years, provides ample opportunity for ongoing connection along the way. In the Tana Toraja regency of South Sulawesi, Indonesia, the bereaved live in close proximity to the deceased's corpse for years. The dead are thought to exist within a liminal phase between life and death and are referred to as merely being *sick* or *asleep*. Family members symbolically feed and care for them. Children play and talk with recently deceased relatives who have been seated in chairs within the home. Torajans often sleep near the dead and keep the corpse close throughout the daytime, often going so far as to carry the body along during important events in the community (Wellenkamp, 1991).

Persisting proximity to corporeal remains gives the bereaved concrete reassurance that some approximation of the dead will continue to be within reach. But others' rituals reanimate the deceased's presence through more abstract and symbolic representations. Japanese culture practices *sosen-suhai*, which translates to *ancestor worship*, a general philosophy about life and death as well as an elaborate system of rituals that convey deep respect for those who have come before. Because the divide between worlds of the dead and the living is considered permeable, the living are able to maintain feelings of closeness with the deceased (Hori, 1994). A beloved family member's spirit is thought to be accessible for approximately thirty-five to fifty years after they pass on, allowing all who knew the deceased to preserve an ongoing bond for the remainder of their own lives.

Most Japanese families maintain an altar to their ancestors, a *butsudan*. Adorned with photographs, cremation ashes, and tablets inscribed with names of the ancestors, these altars are the focal point of rituals that bridge between the world of the living and the world of the dead. And it is from within the humble home that surviving family members reach through the ether to make contact. Family members may evoke the felt presence of the deceased's spirit by lighting candles and clapping hands in front of the butsudan, effectively entering the world of the dead for a short moment. The ritual is then drawn to a close by bowing out and stepping away from the altar, back into the world of the living (Goss & Klass, 2005).

The Obon festival, a cherished annual event, exemplifies the immense value that Japanese culture places on maintaining meaningful ties to the dead. Also known as the Festival of Souls, Obon celebrates the return of the deceased's spirit as worlds of the living and dead briefly merge (Saito, 2014). This Buddhist custom occurs over a span of three days during the autumn equinoxes, when day and night are of equal length and the veil between worlds is at its thinnest. On the first day of the festival, family members visit their ancestors' graves and light lanterns after sunset to guide the spirits back home. The butsudan is cleaned and decorated ahead of time with special lanterns designated for Obon. A welcoming fire is lit at the entrance to the home, where family members gather to formally greet their ancestors upon their return and offer a variety of foods. At the conclusion of the festival, a farewell fire is lit, again at the entrance to the home, and family members visit the grave once more to send off the ancestors' spirits with a spoken invitation to return the following year (Hendry, 2003).

The Japanese Obon festival shares much in common with other cultures whose customs and rituals affirm continuing bonds while simultaneously embracing physical absence. People in the Sanyuan Village of China practice *yingwang anwei* (welcoming back the soul of the dead), during which a priest places a kerosene lamp at the front door of the home to illuminate a path for the deceased to return home, where food and liquor await their arrival. The Mexican holiday of Dia de los Muertos carves out time every year for family members and the community at large to find respite in brief reunion with the souls of their dead. These and many other mourning rituals represent a successful resolution of the rapprochement crisis in mourning, a continual process of encouraging appropriate distance from the deceased while also creating a space and time for the bereaved to return to the deceased and rediscover their presence once more.

The attachment perspective: A case for more presence, and a case for less

Within the bereaved resides an indomitable drive to transcend limitations of reality and preserve a meaningful attachment to one's most cherished relationships. As Parkes (1997) stated, "Part of the problem of bereavement is to find a satisfactory location for the dead for there are few who can accept the idea that they are nowhere" (p. 237). Rather than passively waiting to feel the profound touch of a loved one reaching across planes of existence or sitting idle until culture dictates when the dead can be summoned back, the individual can create personal grief rituals to actively foster continuing bonds on their own terms.

The bereaved regularly turn to their external surrounds to inspire an enduring connection to the dead. This has long been the case for humans throughout history. Lewis-Williams and Pearce (2005) have argued that prehistoric tombs functioned as more than mere burial sites; they also reserved a space for the living to be near the dead and return as needed per their own volition. To this day, the bereaved often choose to visit a cemetery or mausoleum at a convenient time so that they can stay close to those who have passed. An urn placed atop the mantel or a framed picture on a chest of drawers demarcates a specific location in the home where a symbol of the departed can always be found waiting, like a grandfather reliably sitting in his favorite chair. And many will find great meaning in relocating cremation ashes into the elements of nature around them, be it a lot of land that can be revisited; in nearby bodies of water, where the spirit continually sails close to the shore; or in the sky, forever hovering overhead. In similar fashion, the Cree Native Americans believed that the magnificent displays of light shining down from the aurora borealis were actually spirits of their ancestors communicating with the living below (Robinson, 2002).

The bereaved may instead grasp external symbols within their reach that represent the deceased's ongoing presence. When designing a personal grief ritual, each individual has the freedom to incorporate whichever objects provide the most meaningful ties to the attachment figure. Be it a treasured possession that the deceased always held on to, a keepsake that rekindles specific memories of time spent with each other, or items once used to enjoy a hobby, such as a set of golf clubs or cooking utensils, otherwise-inanimate things are imbued with symbolism and help the bereaved feel connected to their loved ones well after death.

Others are contented to find that the deceased remain accessible within the internal recesses of their mind. Be it the subjective experience of holding an imaginary conversation, of feeling the warmth of a departed loved one's company, or of seeking guidance from the dead during challenging circumstances, the deceased's presence resonates even when sitting alone in an empty room. The bereaved continue to receive an approximation of the unique relationship they once enjoyed. But they may also find it meaningful to provide the deceased with attentiveness through expressions of gratitude and updates about living family members. Thus, the subjective experience of continuing bonds is often a two-way street. The Tana Toraja of Indonesia, who recognize an eternal and unbreakable bond between the living and the dead, continue to attend to the dead as an ongoing expression of care, rewrapping their remains and repairing damaged coffins (Rosenblatt, 1997). And Japanese ancestor worship hinges upon the notion that the living's attachment to the dead is reciprocal, a circle of interdependence in which the living provide care for the dead and the dead, in turn, watch over the living (Berentsen, 1983).

Most bereaved individuals are able to construct personal grief rituals that lean upon continuing bonds to cope with loss and resolve the rapprochement crisis of mourning. That is, they manage to untangle themselves from the past while still clasping a few strands of what came before. This is largely the benefit of having a secure attachment style. Equipped with a healthy internal working model (IWM), they regard any desire for an enduring connection to be worth preserving over time. And insofar as they possess object constancy, mental representations of the deceased will be an accessible source of solace, just as the actual attachment once provided tactile comforts and words of reassurance. Illusory interactions, visits to meaningful locations, and holding on to inanimate objects imbued with the deceased's essence all promise to aid the bereaved amid their perilous journey through mourning.

Some, however, do not reap the benefits of continuing bonds so easily. Much of this struggle can be related back to the challenges of having *poor object constancy*, an important and complex concept that requires some clarification. Most people are able to access memories of an attachment figure and feel a sense of ongoing connection even when physically absent. They can conjure up an image of the other and hold it in view. They can hear the other's voice and envisage what they might have to say. The other is felt to be present, albeit within a symbolic realm of the mind. But for those who struggle with poor object constancy, it is difficult to maintain a hold on mental representations of the other when separated. Whether due to situational stresses inherent in grief or more stable factors such as an insecure attachment style, a lack of object constancy further complicates the mourning process, making it even more difficult to derive comfort or a sense of continuity from the fleeting vestiges of a relationship that is no longer physically present.

Some individuals attempt to navigate the mourning process by withdrawing from meaningful connections to the deceased altogether. The past is jettisoned and left behind. Preference is given instead towards managing the stresses of life without the deceased, what Stroebe's dual process model of coping with bereavement refers to as *restoration-oriented stress*. Those with a dismissing attachment style are particularly susceptible to this course of mourning as they exhibit a dearth of conscious thoughts or feelings about whomever they lost. The same IWM that steers them away from healthy reliance upon others will, following a loss, rocket them forward into a novel future untethered to those who came before. And yet quiet yearnings for a touch of familiar bonds from the past may persist, however tenuous they are within the mind. Those who suffer from insufficient continuing bonds benefit greatly from personal grief rituals that foster more ongoing connections and amplify strivings for a subjective sense of closeness to the deceased.

But continuing bonds can be a slippery slope, for one can become too connected to the dead. Where some struggle to hear faint echoes of the deceased before they dissipate, others are deafened by a clanging cacophony of ceaseless chatter. Those with a preoccupied attachment style are uniquely susceptible to struggle with such an all-consuming absorption in ties to the past. Every waking hour seems to be predominated by intense yearnings for reunion. Every thought revolves around memories of time once spent together. Behaviors or relationships unrelated to the deceased are avoided; the preoccupied individual flails as she drowns in loss-oriented stress. As follows, any activity that strengthens ties to the deceased may very well plunge the bereaved deeper into a torment of enduring connection already too pervasive in the mind. These individuals would benefit more from personal grief rituals that confront the reality of loss and absence (discussed previously in Chapter 4) and those that aid in adapting to the restoration-oriented stresses of life without the deceased (to be discussed in the next chapter).

Even the inanimate keepsakes held on to after a loss can contribute to wildly varied courses of mourning. Whether mementoes burden the psyche or offer it relief is contingent upon two factors: the individual's subjective experience of loss as well as what the item represents about the lost relationship. Suppose a family of three siblings is mourning the recent deaths of both parents and have decided to sell the childhood home in which their parents lived until their final days. While walking through the rooms one last time, each sibling is compelled to hold on to a few particularly meaningful items. The youngest son grabs a collection of classic movies from the 1930s and 1940s. The middle daughter selects an assortment of her mother's dresses. The eldest son decides to hold on to his father's medal he received for military service during the Second World War. It is fascinating to consider how each of these objects, seemingly neutral on their own, will inspire myriad thoughts and feelings within each person.

The youngest sibling, who had once bonded with his parents through a mutual love of classic films, is able to create a personal grief ritual through which he derives warm nostalgia from repeated viewings of *Citizen Kane*, *Meet Me in St. Louis*, *North by Northwest*, and *Casablanca*. His parents' collection of movies provides a *positive* continuing bond, a Winnicottian transitional phenomena that eases the pain of adjusting to their absence by recreating an illusory sense of their presence as if watching the classics with his mother and father just as they had done many times before. These types of continuing bonds provide comfort while also confronting a loss for what it plainly is.

The middle daughter, however, suffers a markedly different fate with the heirlooms she holds on to. She preserves her mother's dresses with great care but extracts no joy from doing so. In fact, the dresses soon become a source of worry and unease. She anxiously monitors how well their color and quality of fabric are holding up, all of which distract her from contemplating her mother's actual demise. With no intention of slowly relinquishing her attachment to the dresses, her brooding preoccupation obscures feelings of grief. Mere clothing has morphed into a *linking object*, a fetishized talisman whose physical presence is unconsciously misconstrued as a continuation of external contact with her mother. Objects such as these come to represent a *negative* continuing bond that obstructs conscious acceptance of loss and fails to ease the mourning process in any way.

It is heartbreaking to consider how this woman's struggles to maintain healthy continuing bonds are the result of her simply trying to sustain the loving relationship she had with her mother. Naturally, those who once relished a warm and nurturing attachment wish to savor it further. But we may take for granted that not all continuing bonds hark back to a relationship that was decidedly positive; holding on to inanimate objects in an effort to cope with grief is particularly pernicious for those who had an unhealthy relationship with the deceased. The eldest son's chosen keepsake, the medal his father was awarded for military service, is placed on a shelf in his home with pride, where it presides over conversations about his father's wartime heroics. However, contact with this particular item also stirs up deep feelings of shame. Each glance in its direction echoes haunting memories of his father's criticism and disappointment for opting out of a career in the military, thus failing to follow in his footsteps. Keeping the object near continues to make him feel belittled all over again, as if his father were once more judging him in the present moment. In this respect, proximity to the medal is stoking a negative continuing bond that only perpetuates painful aspects of the relationship he had with his father.

In summary, continuing bonds carry the potential to provide a meaningful and ongoing connection to the deceased during the difficult process of mourning. More than simple recall of fond memories, these illusory experiences of the other's presence continue to guide the living and provide emotional comfort, effectively satisfying attachment needs throughout the life span. It is no surprise that many of the cultural grief rituals still to be discussed center on the importance of strengthening an enduring bond after death. And those interested in creating personal grief rituals may wish to do the same. But all involved in their design should be wary of haphazardly encouraging a sense of presence without understanding the impact it will have on the individual's well-being. Undoubtedly, many will benefit from activities and symbols that promote continuing bonds, but many others will be better off reducing ties to the deceased or eliminating them altogether. Rituals that confirm absence and those that foster presence often go hand in hand and can play a complementary role in the mourning process as long as the individual's experience of grief and mourning does not necessitate an intentional emphasis on one or the other.

Walking with the dead and talking with the dead

Those cultures who conceive of death as a gradual process, who value an ongoing connection to the deceased, are by no means intent on letting the dead linger indefinitely. Fear of being tormented by the perpetual presence of ghosts has inspired the creation of rituals that discourage spirits of the dead from remaining forever in limbo, prodding them to make a decisive departure for the next world. Nonetheless, cultural rituals and customs continue to invite the dead to return and be among the living for brief and delimited intervals before exiting this world again.

The individual may feel a similar pull to actively encourage a sense of the deceased's presence, albeit within parameters that stave off the haunting feeling that a loved one's specter is hovering nearby at all times. Personal grief rituals can be crafted in a manner that carves out time and space for symbolic interactions with the dead, whether through casual conversation, through welcoming their felt presence during a walk, or while engaged in various leisurely activities. It should be noted that these types of rituals, which aim to foster continuing bonds, are markedly different from those discussed in Chapter 4 that find the bereaved talking *about* the deceased or revisiting old stomping grounds so as to acknowledge absence and the passing of time.

Talia, whose husband of fifty-five years died suddenly in his sleep, wanted to resume taking walks early in the morning to enjoy bird-watching, a lifelong hobby of hers, in quietude. But she was stalled. When I asked why she was hesitating, Talia expressed fear that taking walks alone without her husband would only make her feel more lonely. She deserved room within her grief to express the sadness of being separated from Jonathan, as I did not want to quash her upset entirely. Still, I suggested that she might be able to symbolically take her husband with her on these walks in some meaningful way. Talia had her husband's remains cremated and placed in an urn that rested atop Jonathan's old nightstand. Given my prompt, she decided to take a small container of his ashes with her on early-morning jaunts, her "morning walks with Jonathan," as she came to call them. She only carried out this personal grief ritual for a few months. A true act of transitional phenomena, Talia eventually grew content leaving the ashes at home while wandering about in nearby parks to gaze at goldfinches and sparrows.

Let us now consider how a similar type of grief ritual was developed to cultivate continuing bonds through conversation with the dead and other activities while alone. Kiara was a young woman in her early twenties who came in for grief therapy shortly after the death of her older brother, Arnit. Tragic as it was, this loss came as no surprise to anyone who knew him well. Kiara and her family members had watched for more than ten years as Arnit battled an unforgiving addiction to heroin. His struggles were marked by numerous overdoses and subsequent medical interventions to revive him, a few stints in jail, and more cycles of treatment, recovery, and relapse than Kiara could recall. As is often the case with any prolonged illness, her family had ample time to process anticipatory feelings of grief should Arnit eventually succumb to his demons. The reality that his presence would likely leave them in the future had sunk in nearly a decade prior to the funeral. And so on the morning Kiara awoke to a phone call from her father informing her that her brother had died from yet another overdose, she was neither shocked nor overwhelmed. Grief-stricken as she was to lose her brother, she simply called her employer to request time off, packed a bag, and drove eight hours across multiple state lines to mourn with her family.

Kiara returned to Chicago shortly after the funeral and stumbled back into work and her social life. She did not take off any additional time from her job. Nor did she shy away from social gatherings. Nonetheless, coworkers and friends alike began sharing their concerns that something seemed askew. Was she distracted by intense bouts of grief? No. Kiara expressed a healthy range of feelings about her loss without being consumed by upset for any great stretch of time. Was she under the spell of denial, unwilling to face the facts of Arnit's passing? No. She spoke plainly and without reservation about the reality of how her brother lost his life to addiction. Something else was emerging from behind a brittle facade, something that left others sensing that Kiara was in the room with them but not quite there. She regularly lapsed into states of heightened distraction, as if caught in a daydream. Kiara was failing to be engaged with her colleagues during meetings. While out socializing, she would sit by herself and, with a curious smirk on her face, gaze at the rows of liquor bottles behind the bar, rarely breaking away from her reverie to sip the drink in her hand or talk to one of her friends standing nearby.

I, too, began to notice these brief trancelike moments of quiet disconnect while she was in session with me. She did not seem dissociated or checked out in the way that traumatized patients sometimes become devoid of any apparent emotion or lost in distressing memories of the past. Rather, Kiara would abruptly break from our conversation and crane her neck just slightly up towards the ceiling, as if trying to recount the words to a song she once loved, before returning her focus to whatever we had been discussing. I inquired into the content of the daydreams that had emerged following her brother's death. She initially brushed them off as nothing of significance. But as I pressed, she eventually revealed with some embarrassment, "I'm pretending to be with Arnit, wherever he is."

Kiara and her brother had always been close. They played together often in childhood. Throughout adulthood, they spoke over the phone multiple times throughout the week and shared many hobbies and interests. In Arnit's absence, Kiara was retreating into what seemed like another plane of existence and imagining entire interactions with her brother. She felt pulled to play out discussions about how their surviving sister and their parents were doing, current world affairs, or recently published books she thought they would both enjoy. But these fantasies of reunion with her brother were routinely cut short out of concern for what others would think if she remained in reverie for too long. I asked, "Do you ever let yourself interact with him in that way when you are alone?" Kiara and I were both surprised that she had inhibited herself, even when out of the public eye, from fully accessing the content of her daydreams.

We began exploring the possibility of developing personal grief rituals in which she could act upon her wish to feel close to her brother when alone, free from concerns about alienating those with whom she worked and socialized. Kiara had already been assembling a selection of items in one corner of the spare bedroom in her apartment that reminded her of Arnit: photos of them together, a candle he had given her as a gift, and books they had both hoped to eventually read. Also, Arnit had been a talented artist and left behind countless sketches of birds, comic book characters, and vistas of nature that stretched miles out into the horizon; Kiara was happy to have held on to a few of her favorites. Despite the calm these objects inspired, she scarcely spent time near them. The spare bedroom seemed sealed off from the rest of her daily activities, a sarcophagus housing the remains of her relationship with Arnit. I suggested that Kiara consider putting aside time to enter that space, linger for a while, and talk to him without interruption. I dared to add, "It could be a . . . *shrine* of sorts." Kiara appeared to be perturbed by my choice of words, saying, "I'd rather think of it as . . . Arnit's corner."

No more than once or twice a week, Kiara would spontaneously decide to unwind from a long day of work by sitting near Arnit's corner and talking with him about her ever-changing life in the Midwest. These conversations did not necessarily pertain to his absence or discussions of how she missed him. Instead, she afforded herself the opportunity to suspend disbelief and be with him in the present moment. In their childhood, Kiara and Arnit would quietly devour books together in the same room, part of what she attributed to her becoming an avid reader early in life. She recreated that familiar sense of presence by relaxing near the collection of Arnit's items and reading a book, sometimes without uttering a word, and at other times stopping to share a comment about the story's characters and plot. Her personal grief ritual encouraged the very thing she was shamefully trying to evade throughout the day while in the company of others. Buoyed by her unmasked wish to remain connected with her brother, Kiara's daydreams ceased to pull her out of the world in which she still lived.

For the sake of play: Recreating what used to occur

The past beckons the bereaved to revisit. Friends regale each other with stories about those they have lost. Family members stoke the embers of memory with slideshows and shoeboxes filled with old photographs. Bereaved individuals return to meaningful locations of past significance and carry out old traditions to maintain continuity between the past and present. But these simple acts of recollection have the potential to become so much more than an acknowledgment of the passing of time. Those who yearn for ongoing connection to the departed may feel a subtle tug in their heart that pulls them to engage once more in activities the bereaved and deceased once enjoyed together. Personal grief rituals can set aside time to do so with a sense of the other's presence and can be tailored to whatever interactions of old still carry the most meaning. Lucy mourned the death of her father by returning to Wrigley Field just as they had done together so many times. Jason maintained his father's legacy by teaching his son how to fish, and on those occasions when he went out into the water alone, he allowed himself to feel as if there were two fishermen in the boat. Kiara benefited from basking in the illusory experience of reading books in her brother's company à la childhood. As previous means of connection are revived, a template from the past is laid upon the present moment and experienced anew.

Cultural death rituals around the world coax out spirits of the dead so that the living may reunite with their departed loved ones through cherished activities of old. Though an assortment of pastimes are used to entice the dead into making the long journey back home – dancing, sharing updates about family members, playing games – none is more persuasive than the universal appeal of connecting through food. The familiar aromas of a culture's traditional fare play an indispensable role in reuniting the living and the dead, tempting the spirits to re-emerge and be present to dine once again on their favorite cuisine. Like the ephemeral bliss of a good meal, the window of time to bond over food is brief before bidding the dead adieu until the next feast.

Radunitsa, an ancient Slavic festival of the dead, is one such set of rituals that incorporated food to stir the dead and maintain ongoing ties with the living. Traditionally of pagan origin, the festival was held in spring, when nature was reawakening from its own languid slumber. The day would begin with customary visits to family graves, where women and girls put mourning on display with a chorus of weeping. But seeing as how Radunitsa was marked as a day for joy and celebration, sorrow and pain soon gave way to irreverent and boisterous festivities. Participants would drink liquor and share a traditional meal at the cemetery, throwing food and drink onto the ground as offerings to the dead, in hopes that they would feel involved, as if they were once again dining with loved ones amid the day's revelry (Kerrigan, 2017).

Whereas Radunitsa has largely fallen out of practice in the past century, *Dia de los Muertos* reaches back hundreds of years and is still well and alive today in Mexico, the United States, in Latin countries throughout Central America, and across the continent of South America. Dia de los Muertos, as it is recognized today, a holiday and set of rituals that invite the dead to reunite with the living, is the product of Aztec religious beliefs colliding with Catholicism brought over by the Spanish Conquistadors in the early sixteenth century. Catholic traditions of All Souls Day and All Saints Day were effectively merged with Aztec customs into something new. Dia de los Muertos celebrates a time of the year during which the border between the spirit world and the world of the living is believed to dissolve and allow souls of the deceased to cross over and be welcomed back to spend time with loved ones. Surviving family members prepare for the occasion by decorating *ofrendas*, special shrines in the home. The ofrendas are adorned with pictures of the dead and sugar skulls painted with an array of vibrant hues. Upon sunset, mischief descends upon the community as the living embellish colorful outfits with strings of shells that, when shaken, clamor loudly in the streets and near grave sites to rouse the dead and invite their presence yet again (Carmichael & Sayer, 1992).

Souls of the dead return eager to dance, play music, drink, and feast with their loved ones as they did in times past. Family members share meals with the dead at the grave site and leave the deceased's favorite foods atop the ofrendas; flowers may be offered as well. The distinctive scents of pozole, tamales, and mole waft through the air and intermingle with thick plumes of incense smoke. Spontaneous changes in the meandering trails of smoke are seen as a sign that the dead walk among the living, disbursing the air with each movement.

Dia de los Muertos stokes the flames of nostalgia vis-à-vis a sense of the deceased's familiar presence in the current moment. Ritualistic offerings of food recreate interactions in which the living carry on nurturing loved ones and keeping them company. As in others' cultural rituals and traditions, provision of care is a two-way street. The promise of a yearly opportunity to bridge the gap between life and the afterlife and reconnect continues to meet the ever-present attachment needs of the living. Ritualized contact with departed family members uplifts the bereaved and steadies their path through mourning.

The impulse to turn to familiar cuisine as a way to recreate meaningful ties to the dead is ubiquitous. Just as this instinctive response to loss pervades Mexican culture, a trip to the other side of our planet finds the Tana Torajans of Indonesia compelled to continue feeding the dead and the Japanese making offerings of food to their ancestors during the Obon festival. Even when one's culture does not prescribe such rituals, many individuals will act on intuition and include the deceased's spirit in activities centered on eating. It is quite telling that new foods are rarely introduced; previous dining experiences pave the most meaningful path towards continuing bonds. A daughter will find comfort in putting aside time on Mother's Day to bake cookies just like she and her mother used to do together, talking out loud the entire time as if asking her mother what still needs to be added to the batter. While mourning the loss of a lifelong friend, the bereaved will stop into their favorite fast-food restaurant from childhood and order two of the same meal. A family will gather during the holidays and, after wasting away an afternoon in the kitchen cooking meals passed down across generations, proceed to set a place for the deceased at the table. Kiara, whose family was of Indian descent, coped with the anniversary of Arnit's death by making plans to eat a traditional American breakfast of eggs, bacon, fruit, and waffles for dinner that evening. She, her sister, and their parents chose to have this meal not because they were particularly fond of that curious combination of carbohydrates, fat, and sugar but because Arnit loved having "breakfast for dinner" and because her family wished to share a meal with him once again.

An entirely different type of personal grief ritual that fosters an enduring connection involves visiting places where the bereaved and the deceased once spent time together. Per the attachment system, searching behaviors of old are reactivated. But unlike those rituals discussed in Chapter 4 that encourage the bereaved to revisit old haunts for the sole purpose of confirming absence after failing to find them, the bereaved may elect to return to meaningful locations for a vastly different reason: *to succeed in rediscovering the deceased's illusory presence*. Our senses play a key role in unlocking memories tied to familiar spaces, whether indoors or out in nature. The distinctive scents, sights, and noises associated with a particular place recreate some semblance of the other's nearness. Perhaps it was the sound of sitting quietly on a fishing boat at dawn and the singular brilliance of a sunrise that helped Jason summon his father's presence. It may have been the unmistakable roar of a crowd at a ballpark and the smell of cheap beer that coaxed out Lucy's father for one evening.

Javier was in his forties when his sister died from chronic congestive heart failure. We began meeting for psychotherapy soon after. At the beginning of every appointment, he would wander into my office with a shoebox of Polaroid pictures tucked underneath his arm. Javier and I spent the majority of our early work together pulling out one photograph after another and reflecting upon childhood memories of growing up alongside his sister, Rachel. Sorrowful tears were interspersed with laughter as he recalled awkward holiday gatherings, their embarrassing tastes in clothing and fashion from the 1970s, and regular outings with their mother and father to see movies, concerts, and plays.

Of all these childhood experiences, he cherished the memory of watching musical theater with his sister the most. Javier and Rachel grew to love the orchestral scores, the witty banter between actors onstage, and their elaborate costumes. He recalled that they shared a similar sense of humor as children and how, much to the chagrin of their parents, they would try to make each other laugh at inappropriate moments when the dialogue was serious. His favorite memories involved them both muffling the sounds of their giggling during the actors' most dramatic exchanges of love and tragedy. As adults, Javier and Rachel continued to accompany each other to various productions of their favorite shows, both old and new: *Phantom of the Opera*, *Wicked*, *Oklahoma!*, and *The Book of Mormon*. It was their way of keeping in touch despite the demands of work and family life.

Soon after the new year began, the anniversary of Rachel's death was drawing nearer. Javier was befuddled as to how he could acknowledge the significance of that date. He struggled to entertain anything other than putting aside more time to leaf through the shoebox of pictures yet again. Clearly frustrated about what to do, Javier blurted out, "I wish I could just go see a play with her again." I decided to seize that moment and encourage him to go exactly where his intuition was pointing towards, saying, "Perhaps you *could* go and let yourself feel like she is with you." This type of suggestion can truly be hit or miss, with some individuals balking at the idea as nothing more than unadulterated fantasy and denial. But Javier took to the suggestion with enthusiasm. A mischievous smile crept up his face, as if he knew he was bending reality for the sake of play. He put the shoebox aside and began considering which production he would like to go see "with Rachel." Javier found this personal grief ritual to be so deeply meaningful and calming that it became an annual tradition. Every January, he would venture downtown in the depths of a Chicago winter and trek through the cold and darkness to be with his sister again, basking in anticipation of the lights going down, the swell of the pit orchestra accompanying the performance, and the inevitable moment when he and Rachel would have to bite their knuckles to fight back an ill-timed giggle.

Vince, discussed at the beginning of this chapter, was also able to rediscover his wife's presence upon returning to locations where they once spent meaningful time together. He was adapting reasonably well to Sophie's death but sensed that something was missing amid his grief. He felt "empty" without any lasting tie to his wife, a bond too important to simply cleave off and leave behind. He plodded through one day after the next with no sense of what he wanted to do at any given moment or where he wished to go. Vince was surprised to find that this feeling of ennui lifted only when at work while near the very spot where Sophie once sat, including the canary-yellow sweater that was still slumped over her chair. I urged him to consider what it was about being proximal to her desk that filled him with ease. With a bashful smile, he said, "This probably sounds crazy, but it's like she's there with me. I know she isn't actually *there*. It's just . . ." An unmistakable feeling of being moved swept over Vince as his eyes welled up. He smiled and continued, "I feel better when I let myself sort of pretend like she is working near me again." I did my best to reassure Vince that his subjective experience of Sophie's presence was a perfectly healthy expression of grief. But there was, in our estimation, one lingering problem: How could Vince actively create continuing bonds without having to go to work?

In the weeks that followed, we talked about the kinds of things he and his wife once did side by side. We explored the possible ways he could seek out activities again in the places where they once occurred whenever he needed to feel connected to Sophie in the present. Nearly every idea involved time they spent outside enjoying nature. Vince was brimming with a zest for life I had not yet seen from him as he detailed the walks they regularly took through parks, along Chicago's beautiful lakefront, and in nature preserves outside of the city when they needed to step away from the vexations of urban life. During these quick road trips out of town, Vince and Sophie grew fond of rolling the windows down and letting their hands undulate against the passing gusts of wind.

Vince began carving out time to explore parks and nature preserves and to walk along beaches just as he and Sophie had always done together, all with a sense of her footsteps accompanying his own. He found calm in the familiar rustling of leaves and the sight of fog hovering over the lake. Over the years, they had developed quite the knack for identifying interesting rock forms and collecting an assortment of those they found during their excursions. Vince decided that a meaningful addition to his personal grief ritual could include intentionally gathering stones and talking with Sophie about what they discovered together. The more Vince engaged in these walks with his wife, the more he felt reassured that there would always be familiar places he could return to if ever he felt empty or alone.

Embodying a symbolic bond: Using clothing, jewelry, and tattoos to signify the other's presence

South Koreans have recently begun turning away from traditional burials. At just under 39,000 square miles in size (approximately the size of Indiana), and with an ever-growing population, South Korea is becoming one of the most densely populated countries in the world. Available land for interment of the dead is at a premium, leaving bereaved families to incur expensive fees for a burial plot whose use is only temporary; per government decree, the dead must be exhumed from the ground after sixty years to make room for the next generation of burials.

But a creative solution has emerged from this dilemma and given rise to an increasingly popular trend in South Korean mourning practices: The deceased's body is cremated, followed by the compression of ashes into smooth *death beads*, tiny gemlike stones that shine with vibrant hues of purple, blue, and green. Born out of pragmatic considerations, compact remains of the deceased are also providing a sentimental solution to the challenges of grief. The bereaved derive emotional comfort from keeping death beads nearby. Whether in transparent glass containers on display within the home or worn around one's wrist or neck as jewelry, these tiny representations of loved ones are kept close amid the pain of absence (Choi, 2012).

Such practices are not entirely unique to South Korea. Many cultures previously discussed – the ancient Nazca civilization of Peru, the Apayao of the Philippines, the peoples of Kiribati, and the Torajans of Indonesia – keep physical remains of the dead close at hand. And these efforts to create tangible ties to the dead are gaining momentum in recent years. *Cremation jewelry*, made from compressed ashes infused into glass, continues to gain popularity around the world as the bereaved opt to embellish their ankles, fingers, wrists, earlobes, and necklines with meaningful ornaments that aid the mourning process.

The residents of New Orleans, a city hard-hit by gun violence, have created a deeply meaningful ritual that helps them cope with the void left behind after a young life is suddenly ripped away. Walk into a home, a backyard party, or a funeral and you may be surprised to see life-size cardboard cutouts of the deceased standing among surviving friends and family members. Though they are somewhat grainy in appearance, the living are all too willing to look beyond these imperfect representations of the dead. The cutouts are regarded as if just another guest at the celebration. And these two-dimensional photographs of a body that no longer radiates warmth nonetheless manage to comfort the bereaved with a healing sense of presence (Lei & Turner, 2019).

The deceased's body proves to be one of the most potent symbols approximating an ongoing bond. Be it their decomposed remains, cremation ashes, or a pictorial representation of the dead, different peoples are compelled to activate that universal instinct that knows no cultural divide: the impulse to seek out some approximation of the attachment figure's presence. In lieu of cultural experiences that provide meaningful access to the deceased's body, or some derivative of such, the individual intent on fostering a symbolic bond to the dead need look no further than their own neck, arms, torso, or legs!

Tattoos prove to be the preferred method of mourning for many, be it an image of a loved one's likeness or a quote that encapsulates their spirit. This form of body modification simultaneously memorializes the dead and invites public acknowledgment of a loss. But these indelible marks on the body prove to be so much more than a nod to what came before and what will hopefully not be forgotten. The various inks and dyes embedded into the skin also serve a deeper function: Tattoos use personally meaningful symbols to establish a sense of closeness to the departed. Roth (2006) referred to these somatic symbols as *memorial tattoos* that commemorate certain aspects of a deceased attachment figure. Susan Samuel (2010) conducted a series of interviews with research participants who had gotten tattoos after a significant loss. Her findings suggest that a memorial tattoo cues memories about the deceased and is often experienced as a transitional object, a comforting representation of the dead and their ongoing presence.

Personal grief rituals may center on the design of a tattoo that incorporates meaningful symbols to maintain continuing bonds. Many of my bereaved clients have begun therapy sessions showing me their embodied works of art after weeks of conversation about which images or words would provide the most lasting tie to their loved ones. Vince rolled up his sleeve to show me Sophie's favorite line of poetry etched into his forearm. With the skin on his arm still raw, he reported a great feeling of ease knowing that the sound of his wife reading poetry to him would ring in his ear anytime he gazed upon the words. Jocelyn, the young woman who lost her father to a sudden heart attack, chose to get a tattoo of a tape measure symbolizing the handiwork that she and her father bonded over. No sooner had the ink dried than she was already contemplating which home repair project she would take on, saying, "We needed to get back home and measure the insulation for the attic." Kiara and her surviving sister, who lived far apart from each other, made plans to get the same tattoo on their right shoulder: a drawing of a blue jay Arnit had made. As Kiara moved forward in life, she expressed an ongoing desire to bare her shoulder and look in the mirror whenever she needed to feel close to her brother. And with her sister joining in on the ritual, they grew closer despite the many miles between them.

Just as ink deposited beneath the epidermis leaves a visible symbol of the deceased that the bereaved carry with them wherever they roam, various items of clothing and jewelry may be laid atop one's skin to represent proximity to the departed. Hats, boots, and sweaters once belonging to loved ones are worn on special occasions to evoke their original owner's essence. Jewelry is kept close around the neck, in one's earlobe, or on any number of fingers. An amulet may sit in a pocket alongside one's hip, acting as a protective talisman that wards off loneliness. The nearness of one's own body, as well as that which adorns it, becomes the seat of ongoing attachment in personal grief rituals that modify the body or dress it up. And this is perfectly healthy insofar as the symbolic is not conflated with whom it signifies! Tattoos, gemstones, or various garments worn on the body can serve as both reminders of absence while also ensuring that the dead remain nearby.

Consuming the dead: Endocannibalism as a meaningful act of mourning

The earliest generation of psychoanalysts, most notably Sigmund Freud and Karl Abraham, were right to draw attention to the psychological significance of a young child's preoccupation with oral gratification. As Jean Piaget later observed, infants *do* explore their surrounds primarily via their mouths. Ever the intrepid creatures, they bite and gum one object after another, discerning between what in this world should be spat out and should be taken in. At our very core, we are driven by an all-consuming need to incorporate what the world and our most formative relationships have to offer. We hunger for attachment figures to *fill us up* with nourishment, knowledge, and love. It is no surprise, then, that psychoanalysts referred to this early phase of development as having a certain cannibalistic quality. A mother's bodily offerings are greedily lapped up again and again in an insatiable quest to quell emptiness and absorb her essence. Mother and child, fundamentally cooperative in this exchange, form a symbiotic bond as each party basks in the other's company.

Later in life, when an attachment figure has died, the irreversibility of their absence is so noxious and intolerable that it reactivates attachment instincts to draw them nearer through continuing bonds. As Freud (1917) noted in his observations on mourning, the grief-stricken individual adrift in a world that feels empty is compelled to internalize and *take in* a symbolic representation of the deceased attachment figure within the inner spaces of the psyche, augmenting one's very sense of self. A modicum of attachment needs remains accessible as the bereaved allow themselves to feel as if they are now enmeshed with the dead's spirit.

But being with the deceased only in abstraction is an unsatisfactory solution for some. Various peoples throughout history have banded together around a fervent belief that the dead's bodily remains are to be interred not beneath the ground but *within* the bereaved themselves. Yes, some have turned to endocannibalism, the consumption of flesh from deceased members of one's community, as a deeply meaningful act of mourning. Such *feasts of the dead* serve multiple functions, but there is perhaps no stronger pull than the wish to forge an ongoing connection between the deceased and the living by collapsing the boundaries between one's own body and that of the other's.

The Wari, a civilization that thrived amid the Andes mountains and along the coast of Peru from AD 600–1000, practiced endocannibalism to ensure that the deceased lived on through fellow tribe members. Graham (2004) has noted that the Wari also believed that consumption of the dead effectively severed one's earthly relationship with the departed. They apparently held an understanding of *absence-and-presence*, the nuanced and dialectical balance between relinquishing an external relationship while also maintaining internal bonds. After the death, the bereaved were permitted two to three days for crying and eulogizing before the deceased's body was roasted in preparation for consumption (Conklin, 2001). Public mourning officially ended with a hunt and a feast to acknowledge that the dead had become one with the animal world and its spirits.

Just north in the Mesoamerican region of North America, and only a few centuries after the Wari civilization collapsed, the Aztecs regularly participated in ritualized cannibalism per their belief that consuming the dead kept their spirit and memory alive in the bodies of the living. And all the way on the other side of the world, the Fore people of Papua New Guinea only recently ceased such practices. They had long held that ritualistic cannibalism helped the living absorb a loved one's life force and maintain a permanent relationship with their spirit. In an ironic twist, these life-affirming efforts actually caused people to die from a strange neurological illness called *kuru* that resulted from ingesting the deceased's brains (Neufeldt, 2012).

Despite increased awareness of its health risks, funerary cannibalism has not been entirely eradicated from the world. The Yanomami tribe, an indigenous people living in the Amazon rain forest of Brazil, still consumes their dead. All members of the community are expected to partake in an important ritual during which they eat a mixture of cremated ashes and a paste consisting of mashed bananas. According to Kenneth Iserson (1994), the Yanomami eat their loved ones' remains primarily to protect them, as they are concerned that the soul will otherwise remain forever in limbo between the worlds of the living and the dead during its liminal metamorphosis. Upon devouring the ashes, the living find comfort in the belief that the deceased's soul has been provided safe harbor until it can eventually be liberated and transition to the spiritual world. The Yanomami are not alone in their motive to protect the dead. Neufeldt (2012) clarifies that, for the Wari, endocannibalism within the community was seen as a compassionate alternative to interring dead loved ones in the cold ground. And the Fore, too, ate their dead in preference to the dearly departed being consumed slowly by worms.

We should resist the pull of incredulity and shock upon discovering that certain tribes have consumed the dead as an act of mourning. There is actually plenty of room for sympathy. Who among us can say they have never managed the inner turmoil of grief and absence by imbibing food, alcohol, or any other substance as a substitute for the relational comforts that once filled us with love? Despite the surprising ubiquity of mourning by way of the mouth, it seems that gorging our bellies to counter feelings of emptiness is doomed to either infect the tribe with kuru or bury emotions beneath a haze of sugars and intoxication. Thankfully, cultural grief rituals abound with alternative, more symbolic efforts to internalize the dead.

Identification: Collapsing boundaries between self and the other

In 1942, a devastating fire blazed through Boston's Cocoanut Grove nightclub at an alarmingly fast pace, killing approximately 492 people in a matter of minutes. Erich Lindemann (1944), a psychiatrist specializing in bereavement, interviewed grieving family members so as to study the symptomology of trauma and grief. He observed and documented many common reactions to loss: somatic distress, preoccupation with an image of the deceased, unfounded guilt relating to the circumstances, hostility, and an inability to resume previous levels of functioning. But Lindemann also noted something less common and quite peculiar in many of the survivors' behaviors: They spontaneously began to adopt traits and behaviors once possessed by their loved ones while still alive. Lindemann called this phenomenon *identification*. The bereaved might find themselves altering their gait and walking like the deceased. They would suddenly take interest in the deceased's hobbies and other daily activities. Some even reported seeing resemblances to those they had lost staring back at them in the mirror. How can we make sense of such a curious response to loss, grief, and mourning?

Albert Bandura's (1977) *social learning theory* begins with the simple observation that children mimic adaptive behaviors modeled by important relational figures. Further, the theory argues that children will continue to embody these acquired mannerisms if repeatedly reinforced. A father uses humor to connect with others, and the child within earshot shares his newfound arsenal of jokes with friends to make them laugh. A mother calms her infant with a gentle tone of voice, and the older child is applauded upon echoing her mother's soothing words when talking to her younger sibling. Social learning theory is a well-established set of observations about human behavior. Nonetheless, it leaves much to be desired in our efforts to understand why the bereaved might take on traits of the deceased *only after they have passed*.

Joseph Weiss (1993) viewed identification through the lens of attachment theory. He posited that children are unconsciously motivated to identify with attachment figures so as to maintain a symbolic union that mollifies primitive fears of disconnect and separation, not unlike how infants are compelled to crawl closer to loved ones. To *be like* someone is to feel close to them. Telling jokes as father does or comforting the youngest sibling in a manner similar to mother produces a reassuring sense of kinship between self and the attachment figure.

The subjective experience of incorporating another person's fundamental characteristics into one's own identity and somehow feeling fused in the process accentuates how permeable are the boundaries that demarcate self from the other. Identity encompasses a constellation of behaviors, thoughts, feelings, social roles, and attributes that correspond to the kind of person one essentially is across varying contexts. But these qualities do not crystallize into an immutable self that is sealed off from other people. Identity evolves and remains open to the ongoing influence of important relationships throughout the life span. We not only identify with those we relate to, in whom we already see a bit of ourselves, but also identify with those we wish to emulate. We adapt to be more like whomever we love and admire. The manner in which the other articulates themselves, masters a skill, or maintains a cool head when under pressure is internalized as a goalpost to aim for, and upon aligning one's own behaviors with the other, they are felt to be *with us* in a sense.

Sidney Blatt's (2006) research on personality configurations gives us pause to contemplate the dialectical relationship between *self-definition* and *relatedness*. Only if we are fully aware of ourselves as being different from others (self-definition) can we use empathy to comprehend another person's separate experience (relatedness). At the same time, interactions with others inform who we are, leaving us utterly dependent upon relationships to define our individual sense of self. And the psychoanalytic concept of a *selfobject* tells us that others are experienced as extensions of our own sense of self: In the mother's approving gaze lies our confidence; our friend's laughter becomes our joy. The self is fundamentally enmeshed with others.

Returning again to Susan Samuel's (2010) research, she found that memorial tattoos usually begin as a symbol that represents the deceased but often become introverted and experienced as a part of the self. When participants were asked to comment on what it would be like if their tattoo were suddenly erased, many stated that it would feel like a missing limb, like a part of themselves would be gone, and that the tattoo could not simply be replaced with another. Representations of the other came to merge with the self in an effort to heal from loss and cope with absence.

Certain pangs of grief make it all too apparent that one's sense of self is intimately tethered to important relationships. The bereaved regularly report a state of internal emptiness while in mourning, a vacuum of great uncertainty where once there was a solid shape and form to whom one essentially is. In an effort to make meaning out of life as it moves forward without a once-crucial relationship, one may find themselves asking, *Who am I in light of this loss?* or, *What is my role or responsibility in what has come to pass?* (Neimeyer & Thompson, 2014). *Who am I,* the bereaved wonders, *if no longer someone's spouse, if they cannot attend religious services with their mother anymore, or if not joined at the hip to a lifelong friend?* Loss guts identity, the natural response being to reactivate the attachment system and mobilize searching behaviors to fill the void. But with what?

Identification is one such tactic. As an act of protest, one can cushion the fall into absence by rediscovering a loved one through alterations to his or her own sense of self! The lasting influence of the departed still remains accessible, albeit within the bereaved individual's adopted behaviors, utterances, and values. Indeed, Horowitz (1990) asserted that *the mental schema of attachment must be revised in order to accommodate the reality of loss,* and Field (2006) added, "Such revision may encompass change in the representation of the self through internalization of valued attributes of the deceased into the ego-ideal" (p. 741).

Cultures located far from one another have intuitively used this solution to guide themselves through mourning and ultimately arrive at the same destination; their customs and grief rituals remedy the problem of loss by encouraging identification with the deceased. In Jewish tradition, the Kaddish prayer of mourning is considered to be a means by which the bereaved now acts as a mouthpiece for the dead, thus creating a sense of identification. Anniversaries are also considered to be a time of the year for surviving family members to perpetuate the dead's legacy with good deeds (Levine, 1997). Muslim tradition encourages those who knew the deceased well to relay stories of their most noble behaviors so as to inspire the living to embody those very qualities, memorializing the dead not only in words but also through action (Philips, 2005). Such identification is thought to create continuing bonds. Performing good deeds or giving to charity in the name of the dead provides opportunities to retreat into nostalgia via storytelling and simultaneously create a present-day symbolic representation of the dead. It is also customary to hang pictures of the dead within one's home and to breathe new life into the deceased's legacy by naming children after them. Muslims traditionally put aside three days for a formal period of mourning, but efforts to identify with the dead persist well beyond their final days (Yasien-Esmael & Rubin, 2005).

Australia's Aboriginal people have a rich history replete with unique rituals designed to keep departed loved ones near in both body and spirit. Though a given community may eventually cremate the dead or bury their remains, tradition still dictates that the corpse is to be left outside and hoisted high above the ground onto an elevated platform, where it will decompose. Surviving family members cover the body with leaves and branches and then show great patience as they wait for time and decay to strip the corpse of all but its skeleton. Bereaved family members eventually return to collect the bones, paint them with red ochre, and may even carry or wear the bones for up to a year. Specific to the Moranoa people of Australia, a centuries-old tradition involves collecting liquid from a smoked and desiccated corpse and rubbing it over the bodies of young men so as to pass on good qualities of the deceased to the living (Howitt, 1907).

These culturally prescribed rituals highlight how crucial it is for the bereaved to understand the meaning behind any act of mourning. Muslims knowingly take on the deceased's best traits to sustain an ongoing bond beyond death. The Moranoa are fully aware of why liquids seeping out of the dead are to be absorbed into their own skin. But plenty of individuals swept up in the swirling tempests of mourning are thrown this way and that by forces that confound them. Lindemann's research was all the more fascinating in that many who found themselves identifying with the deceased did so unintentionally. If identification occurs outside of one's conscious awareness and willful choice, the bereaved may take on traits they wish they would not or remain confused and unable to find meaning in the way their loved one's personality suddenly reverberates throughout their own. This aligns with what Steven Foreman (2018) dubbed *pathological identification*, "a learned, psychological phenomenon in which a person unconsciously repeats or reenacts problematic behaviors, feelings, attitudes, relationship patterns or dilemmas exhibited by significant others, usually parents, in the past" (p. 15). Common examples include ineffective behaviors that lead to failure at work or in relationships, poor emotional regulation, self-defeating attitudes, and substance abuse.

Lydia's befuddling manifestation of grief exemplifies how *unconscious, pathological identification can beget complicated bereavement*. Following her father's death from a protracted battle with leukemia, Lydia found herself drinking tequila alone on work nights. The setting and sequence were always the same. She would stay up well into the morning hours, nursing one libation after another, while listening to the radio in her kitchen. Its blown speakers crackled with the rhythms of samba, merengue, and salsa music, all to the chagrin of her wife, who had to wake up early for work. Lydia was baffled by her behavior. The recurrent hangovers and lack of sleep made for grueling workdays, but she was truly mystified by her behavior because she *did not enjoy drinking alcohol*! Such uncharacteristic indulgence was written off as no more than a run-of-the-mill attempt to drown grief in booze. However, as we continued to dig for clues about the meaning of this behavior, we unearthed something much more specific to her relationship with her father.

Lydia reminisced about childhood memories of her father's long work hours and the sparse opportunities she had to spend time with him after his shifts. She recalled many instances of being woken up in the middle of the night by a series of loud noises. Lydia, only nine years old, would walk out of her room to find her father drinking tequila . . . and listening to Latin music on the radio . . . in the kitchen . . . to the chagrin of Lydia's mother! She and I agreed that behaving akin to her father in his absence represented an unconscious pull to feel close to him vis-a-vis identification. With the implicit function of her behaviors laid bare, Lydia thirsted for tequila no more, and we were then able to discuss healthier and more fulfilling ways by which she could identify with her father.

Any individual hoping to establish greater continuing bonds may find that mimicking the deceased's behaviors is the preferred route to take. But as Lydia's plight makes evident, acts of identification lend themselves to healthy expressions of mourning only insofar as they are enacted with conscious awareness. Thus, this type of personal grief ritual should provide an opportunity to articulate the meaning behind specific acts of behavioral mimicry prior to their performance.

Recall Matthew from the previous chapter. His sister's death left him struggling to cope during meaningful dates and holidays. But with the help of personal grief rituals that put aside time to feel what had been kept numb, he managed to traverse a year of firsts without his sister's company and truly mourn his loss. He and his family spent countless hours during that first year sharing stories and reminiscing about the sister, daughter, mother, and aunt they lost. Nonetheless, Matthew still missed his sister dearly, saying, "I feel so distant from her." The mere retrieval of memories and shedding of tears did not quite scratch what was itching. He wanted to somehow feel, as he said, "connected" to his sister in the present moment.

I asked Matthew to think about anything he could do that might help him feel closer to his sister, perhaps something that would capture the essence of who she was or embody what she liked to do in her spare time. He recalled a fleeting thought that occurred to him many times over the past few months. Matthew's sister had quite the green thumb; she enjoyed gardening and had a particular penchant for sunflowers. He had frequently entertained the idea of planting sunflower seeds at numerous locations – in his backyard, at a park near his work, along the streets of his neighborhood – before quickly disregarding it as a useless whim. Rather than truncate the thought, we sustained our focus on the meaning of this fantasy. Matthew's eyes gleamed with a tranquil glow as he relished the prospect of "doing something she would do." His loneliness seemed to ease a bit as he began setting aside time to plant sunflower seeds and feel close to his sister.

The Bara of Madagascar believe that we live not in repeated cycles of rebirth like the waxing and waning moon but instead like the tree passing on its legacy through seeds that fall to the ground and spring up into new life (Metcalf & Huntington, 1991). People all around the world identify with those they have lost by using their very sense of self to harvest memories of the dead and breathe new vitality into the seedlings left behind. The bereaved are the stewards of legacy. But time, red in tooth and claw, aims to devour personal history and render entire lives forgotten and irrelevant. Personal grief rituals that center on identifying with the dead ensure that the past is kept alive and well, preserving a comforting link to the past that accompanies the living as they venture ahead into a world the deceased never traversed.

Treading where the dead never roamed

It had been six years since Libby first stepped into my office after her mother died from brain cancer. The bulk of our work together had focused on excavating all that was now behind her. Libby felt her way through one loss-oriented feeling of grief after another. She reflected on all that she wished were still present in her life: childhood memories of riding bikes with her mother, frequenting bookstores together in adulthood, and regular phone calls to lament about the stresses of early parenthood. She steadily confronted the reality of her loss, and still, she yearned to remain connected to her mother. We developed various personal grief rituals that blocked off chunks of time for her to return to meaningful places and recreate activities they once enjoyed together. Libby rode her bike down familiar paths near her childhood home on the weekends. She basked in the quietude of her mother's favorite bookstore and read a new novel while drinking coffee just like they had done many times, even as her mother was fighting fatigue from radiation treatments.

But opportunities to breathe new life into cherished memories of old began to fade beyond her reach. Libby and her siblings finally sold the house in which they grew up, where her mother spent her last days while receiving hospice care. Libby, her husband, and their two children packed up their own home and moved to a new neighborhood where there were no well-traveled bike paths nearby and no local bookstores filled with nostalgia. Libby's life had pulled her further away from remnants of her mother's life. Prior to taking a family vacation to France and Italy, she ended her appointment saying, "I just don't feel her with me anymore."

Libby returned from her time abroad and reported a most curious event. While sightseeing, she was repeatedly overcome with an unmistakable feeling that her mother was experiencing it all with her, viewing tourist attractions, as she put it, "through my eyes." Standing beneath the Arc de Triomphe, Libby and her mother gazed down the magnificent tree-lined streets of the Champs-Elysees stretching deep into the heart of Paris. They walked among the ruins of Pompeii together and stared at Mount Vesuvius in the distance with quiet awe. Libby mourned her mother's absence amid reminders that she was no longer able to explore the wonders of the world, something she had held out hope for resuming once treatment was complete. At the same time, this illusory sense of her presence, as if bringing her mother along to see the world for herself, left her overjoyed. Libby began considering how to design entirely different types of personal grief rituals through which she could explore bike paths and bookstores where her mother never treaded but without leaving her entirely behind.

Doing what the deceased *never did* represents a unique expression of continuing bonds in part because it is a gross departure from the past. There are no footprints to retrace when treading where the deceased never journeyed. A symbolic mental representation of the dead can accompany the bereaved as they experience something new, but the individual who steps into territory uncharted by the deceased simultaneously cements the poignant truth that a loved one is no longer able to participate in life. The emotional content of such rituals is often overwhelmingly bittersweet, especially if the chosen activity involves something the bereaved had hoped to do with their loved one before they died.

A personal grief ritual that finds the bereaved experiencing life anew may prove to be heart-wrenching, but such novel sojourns facilitate mourning by affirming a deep and quiet desire to resume living a life of excitement and adventure that is only loosely tethered to the past. It is beyond coincidence that *many choose to go somewhere new as a meaningful act of mourning*, even as they maintain continuing bonds along the way. Libby put aside time to be with her mother while visiting exotic locations far from home that she and her mother had longed to see together. Vince built upon the initial grief ritual he created and began seeking out spots in nature he and his wife never explored together. A small glass container filled with her cremated ashes accompanied him on every such journey; whenever he sauntered down an unfamiliar walking path in a wooded area he thought Sophie might have enjoyed, he would spread some of her ashes near a tree, beneath a rock, or in a small body of water, "so she can experience how beautiful it all is."

Let us return to the case of Tameeka, the woman whose selection of a mauve dress evoked complex feelings about her mother's death. Our initial work together concluded as she was readying herself to move to Santa Fe for work. Three years had passed when I received an email again from Tameeka.

She was planning to visit her family in Chicago on two separate occasions over the summer and was hoping to schedule a therapy appointment both times she was back in town. I was intrigued to hear how she had been doing and was teeming with questions. Was she adjusting to life in New Mexico? Were any of her initial struggles with grief lingering years after her loss? Had she resumed wearing bright colors to work events?

Upon returning to my office, Tameeka expressed concerns that she was no longer able to conjure up positive memories of her mother since leaving Chicago. With no sense of her mother's presence in a city they had never explored together, Tameeka felt unmoored. Her mother was absent in her external surrounds and, subsequently, within her mind as well. But back in Chicago, her homecoming renewed a swell of continuing bonds everywhere she went: the church at which she and her mother worshipped, the home where she was raised, and the clothing stores they frequented together. Each of these places revived memories of her mother's lasting impact and the nearness of her within Tameeka's heart. But when situated in a corner of the world where no memories had ever been forged, where could she go to sound the echoes of her mother's voice and find a trace of her ongoing presence?

Tameeka and I spent the remainder of that first appointment considering how she could create continuing bonds by doing what she and her mother once did together, albeit in a new city where her mother had never been. She quickly landed on the possibility that she could explore clothing stores near her new home *with her mother*. Tameeka took great pleasure in anticipating the opportunity to check out novel fashions from Santa Fe that neither she nor her mother had ever tried. Most importantly, she gave herself permission in advance to evoke her mother's voice and let herself be goaded into buying nice clothes that made her feel confidant while conducting business. Two weeks later, Tameeka returned to Chicago beaming with excitement. She spent the entire appointment talking about how fulfilling it was to bring her mother with her while shopping in Santa Fe, saying, "It was like she was with me again."

Libby, Vince, and Tameeka each implemented a unique personal grief ritual that attests to the power of creating enduring connections to the dead. Specifically, they each sought out new and enriching experiences made more meaningful by a subjective sense that their departed loved ones were at their side to experience such novelties with them. This type of ritual certainly deserves consideration as a component of healthy mourning. But the prospect of present-day life being enveloped in illusory ties to past attachments invites us to revisit a familiar conundrum: At what point in time after a loss would it be best for the bereaved to move forward and experience life anew free from the deceased's presence? Under what circumstances would it be more advisable to explore new cities, forests, and fashion boutiques without bringing the dead along?

The journey behind and what lies ahead: Where, in time, do the dead belong?

The bereaved dance with a corpse in Madagascar. In Japan, earthbound descendants of the dead hold court with their ancestors. And in the United States, a widowed woman clasps a jar of her husband's ashes while enjoying an early-morning walk in solitude. These subjective encounters with the other's presence, whether by means of a cultural death rite or personal grief ritual, regularly prove to be self-corrective as they slowly usher in acknowledgment of loss and spur the bereaved to move forward with life.

Many cultural conceptualizations of death patiently invite an extended phase of mourning. Death slithers towards its prey at a painstakingly slow pace, fangs drawn and ready for the inevitable kill. But prior to its definitive bite, reoccurring ceremonies maintain meaningful ties between the deceased and bereaved in the liminal interim. Any wish for reunion is acknowledged alongside an understanding that the ritual will end; the unforgiving automaton of death finally comes to collect its due for the loan of life, and all parties must pay the debt. As the spirit gradually relinquishes its earthly body before being fully incorporated into the afterlife, so, too, must the bereaved gradually step away from what came before and courageously walk into a new life.

Continuing bonds maintain an integral role in a healthy response to loss, even after mourning draws to a close and the bereaved begin to decisively move forward beyond an acute state of grief. Such metamorphosis among the living is paralleled by various cultural perceptions of the dead evolving over time, ultimately arriving at its own resolute state of change. The Tana Torajans' customs embrace a prolonged phase of liminality as the living continue to interact with bodily remains of the dead as if still alive. And though they will persist in maintaining a meaningful bond with their loved ones for months or years, a massive and expensive funeral eventually acknowledges the true finality of death. During the Obon festival in Japan, it is believed that spirits of the recently deceased loosen their ties to the living at the end of their first Obon. They are repeatedly called back home to be with the living during each year's celebrations, only to be sent away again after the third day of festivities to resume their long spiritual journey, the goal of which is to transform over time from human spirits (*shirei*) to godly *kami* (Saito, 2014).

Winnicott's notion of transitional phenomena highlights how people cope with separation, and even death, by clinging to a symbolic representation of whoever is absent. Be it a mental representation of the attachment figure or an inanimate item that stands in for the other's nearness, a subjective experience of presence cushions the fall into the harsh reality of grief and mourning. *But the object is not necessarily held on to in perpetuity.* Winnicott (1953) gave equal consideration to the importance of eventually relinquishing the transitional object that signifies what has been lost, saying:

> Its fate is to be gradually allowed to be decathected, so that in the course of years it becomes not so much forgotten as relegated to limbo. By this I mean that in health the transitional object does not "go inside" nor does the feeling about it necessarily undergo repression. It is not forgotten and it is not mourned. It loses meaning.
>
> (p. 91)

Thus, transitional phenomena denote an intermediary point of liminality between separation and eventual efforts to recalibrate to life after a loss.

For those cultures who incorporate the deceased's actual body into death rites and rituals, the corpse itself functions as a transitional object. Surviving family members and loved ones continue to interact with the corpse in many ways just the same as when the deceased was alive. Nonetheless, death dawns on the bereaved with ever greater certainty as the body decomposes, a symbol of ongoing connection that decays and loses meaning over time until the final corporeal remains are interred for good during ceremonial secondary burials. And the individual who incorporates symbols of continuing bonds into personal grief rituals may need to abandon these representations of the deceased in due time. Holding on indefinitely to a semblance of a lost relationship can be beneficial for some, but it is advisable for others to sail into the future unanchored to the past.

Vince continued to venture farther away from the home he had shared with Sophie to explore remote nature preserves they never explored together. A small pouch of Sophie's ashes accompanied him each time he took a long drive out of the city to be with her. Two years had passed, and though this personal grief ritual persisted, its frequency waned as he was less and less in need of an illusory connection to her. Vince's life began opening up in surprising ways. He made new friends. He cultivated novel hobbies. And approximately two and a half years after Sophie's death, Vince fell in love with someone new.

The third wedding anniversary since Sophie's death was fast approaching, and Vince had been feeling pulled to relinquish his solitary trips into the woods. I proposed that we make a slight variation to his regular ritual, one that would entail exploring somewhere new but without bringing her along. Naturally, Vince was torn, but he genuinely felt that Sophie had kept him company on enough adventures after her death. He felt it was time to walk into the future without her at his side. On the date of their wedding anniversary, he visited the church where they got married and spread her ashes one last time. Vince then proceeded to go camping for an extended weekend. He told me that he commemorated the trip by driving out of the city with the windows down, just as he and Sophie had always done, feeling the breeze rush over his outstretched hand and across the tattoo that decorated his arm. A few months later, during what proved to be our last appointment, Vince walked into my office with a joyous smile and informed me that he proposed to his girlfriend and was now engaged.

Embedded within fairy tales, ancient myths, and contemporary movies, long-held truths emerge about how the bereaved must reconcile the pull of old and familiar comforts with the allure of exploring an unknown future. It is no accident that our most cherished stories are replete with tales of deceased loved ones and the aftermath that leaves our hero chained to the past, afraid to take on what lies ahead. I have long been captivated by the movie *Up*, a story that I believe depicts the importance of creating personal grief rituals that explore what remains of one's life while bringing the dead along for the journey -- if only to eventually let them go.

The story begins with a charming tale of how Carl and the love of his life, Ellie, met at a young age. They quickly bonded over their mutual excitement about one day visiting Paradise Falls, a remote waterfall hidden deep in the rain forests of South America. Throughout childhood, and well into their marriage, they save every spare nickel and dime in hopes of one day taking the trip of a lifetime. But fate deters their plans as Ellie succumbs to illness. Carl, now an old and widowed man, roots himself to the house in which they lived and sits in bitter grief, stubbornly refusing to move despite the cacophonous noises of construction reverberating around his home.

Circumstances force him to uproot from his lot of land. But in one final act of rebellion, he rips their home out from the ground with an absurd bulk of balloons and ascends skyward, en route to finally see Paradise Falls for himself and on behalf of his dear wife. Carl speaks to the house throughout his journey as if it were Ellie herself. He turns to her for comfort when distressed as a host of misfortunes besets him and threatens to thwart their path. Later in the story, Carl discovers a message that Ellie wrote him at the end of her life encouraging him to move forward and seek out new adventures without her. The house, having accompanied him into uncharted territory, and into a new friendship with a neighborhood boy named Russell, finally slips away into the clouds beyond his reach. But Carl remains at peace as his journey concludes. The last shot of the movie reveals that the house landed at its intended destination. Ellie, it seems, had transcended to her final resting place, and the audience is left satisfied knowing that Carl is continuing to live his life anew.

References

Bandura, A. (1977). *Social learning theory*. Prentice-Hall.

Berentsen, J. M. (1983). The ancestral rites in missiological perspective. *Japanese Religions*, *13*(1), 2–27.

Blatt, S. J. (2006). A fundamental polarity in psychoanalysis: Implications for personality development, psychopathology, and the therapeutic process. *Psychoanalytic Inquiry*, *26*(4), 494–520.

Carmichael, E., & Sayer, C. (1992). *The skeleton at the feast: The Day of the Dead in Mexico*. University of Texas Press.

Choi, J. Y. (2012, January 21). South Korea firm turns human ashes into beads. *Los Angeles Times*. www.latimes.com/world/la-xpm-2012-jan-21-la-fg-south-korea-death-beads-20120122-story.html
Conklin, B. A. (2001). *Consuming grief: Compassionate cannibalism in an Amazonian society*. The University of Texas Press.
Field, N. (2006). Unresolved grief and continuing bonds: An attachment perspective. *Death Studies*, *30*, 739–756.
Foreman, S. A. (2018). Pathological identification. *Psychoanalytic Psychology*, *35*(1), 15–30.
Freud, S. (1917). Mourning and melancholia. *Standard Edition*, *14*, 243–258. Hogarth Press.
Goss, R., & Klass, D. (2005). *Dead but not lost: Grief narratives in religious traditions*. AltaMira Press.
Graham, H. (2004). Endo-cannibalism in the making of a recent British ancestor. *Mortality*, *9*(3), 255–267.
Hendry, J. (2003). *Understanding Japanese society*. Routledge.
Hori, I. (1994). *Folk religion in Japan: Continuity and change*. Chicago University Press.
Horowitz, M. J. (1990). A model of mourning: Change in schemas of self and others. *Journal of the American Psychoanalytic Association*, *38*, 297–324.
Howitt, A. (1907). The native tribes of south-east Australia. *The Journal of the Royal Anthropological Institute of Great Britain and Ireland*, *37*, 268–278.
Iserson, K. V. (1994). *Death to dust: What happens to dead bodies*? Galen Press, Ltd.
Kerrigan, M. (2017). *The history of death*. Amber Books.
Lei, C., & Turner, T. (2019, January 14). *They still take pictures with them as if the person's never passed*. NPR: The Picture Show. www.npr.org/sections/pictureshow/2018/07/20/630799667/life-size-cutouts-help-extend-the-relationship-with-lost-loved-ones-in-new-orlea
Levine, E. (1997). Jewish views and customs on death. In P. Laungani & W. Young (Eds.), *Death and bereavement across cultures* (pp. 98–130). Routledge.
Lewis-Williams, J. D., & Pearce, D. G. (2005). *Inside the Neolithic mind: Consciousness, cosmos, and the realm of the gods*. Thames & Hudson.
Lindemann, E. (1944). Symptomatology and management of acute grief. *American Journal of Psychiatry*, *101*(2), 141–148.
Metcalf, P., & Huntington, R. (1991). *Celebrations of death: The anthropology of mortuary ritual*. Cambridge University Press.
Neimeyer, R. A., & Thompson, B. E. (2014). Meaning making and the art of grief therapy. In B. E. Thompson & R. A. Neimeyer (Eds.), *Grief and the expressive arts: Practices for creating meaning* (pp. 3–13). Routledge.
Neufeldt, R. (2012). Biasing cannibalism in anthropology. *Journal of Manitoba Anthropology*, *30*, 1–7.
Parkes, C. M. (1997). Conclusions II: Attachments and losses in cross-cultural perspective. In P. Laungani & W. Young (Eds.), *Death and bereavement across cultures* (pp. 233–242). Routledge.
Philips, A. A. B. (2005). *Funeral rites in Islam* (2nd ed.). International Islamic Publishing House.
Robinson, D. B. (2002). *The Cree of North America*. Lerner Publications Co.
Rosenblatt, P. C. (1997). Grief in small-scale societies. In P. Laungani & W. Young (Eds.), *Death and bereavement across cultures* (pp. 27–51). Routledge.
Roth, D. (2006). Adornment as a method of interior design. *Studies in Gender and Sexuality*, *7*(2), 179–194.
Saito, C. (2014). Engaging in grief ministry in multireligious contexts. *Pastoral Psychology*, *63*(1), 105–112.

Samuel, S. A. (2010). *An examination of the psychological role of tattoos in mourning* (Publication No. 3436691) [Doctoral dissertation, The Chicago School of Professional Psychology]. ProQuest Dissertations Publishing.

Talu, A. (1998). *Kiribati: Aspects of history.* Institute of Pacific Studies and Extension Services, University of the South Pacific, and Ministry of Education, Training and Culture, Kiribati Government.

Vanoverbergh, M. (1939). *The Isneg life cycle: Marriage, death and burial.* Catholic Anthropological Conference.

Weiss, J. (1993). *How psychotherapy works.* Guilford Press.

Wellenkamp, J. C. (1991). Fallen leaves: Death and grieving in Toraja. In D. R. Counts & D. A. Counts (Eds.), *Coping with the final tragedy: Cultural variation in dying and grieving* (pp. 113–134). Baywood Publishing Company.

Winnicott, D. W. (1953). Transitional objects and transitional phenomena – A study of the first not-me possession. *The International Journal of Psychoanalysis, 34,* 89–97.

Worden, J. W. (2008). *Grief counseling and grief therapy: A handbook for the mental health practitioner* (4th ed.). Springer Publishing Company.

Yasien-Esmael, H., & Rubin, S. S. (2005). The meaning structures of Muslim bereavements in Israel: Religious traditions, mourning practices, and human experience. *Death Studies, 29*(6), 495–518.

Chapter 7

Moving forward

Rituals that embrace new life

Karol flashed a nervous smile upon entering my office for her first appointment. She sat down on the couch and gripped her knees, as if holding herself down for fear that she would float away. A middle-aged woman in her early fifties, Karol was coming to therapy to discuss a raft of losses she had accrued throughout life, each of which generated a stream of daily reminiscences about the relationships she once enjoyed. Her father passed when she was in her twenties; she had been his primary caregiver for three years during the end of a fifteen-year battle with Alzheimer's disease. She lost two colleagues quite suddenly in her thirties, one in a tragic accident, the other in a violent chance encounter with gang gunfire. She had also been thinking much lately of her friend Samantha, whom she met in a cancer recovery group while in her early forties. Karol remained in remission over the decade that had passed since forging their friendship. Samantha, however, had relapsed in recent years and ultimately died a few days before Karol turned fifty years old. Her fifty-first birthday was only weeks away.

As I asked her to tell me more about her relationship with Samantha, Karol's gaze shot up, almost inward towards her own mind, seemingly scanning her thoughts to ensure the memories remained intact. She then said, "I worry I'm going to forget her. I worry I'll forget them *all* one day!" I asked her what she hoped to accomplish in grief therapy. She responded, "I just want to make sure I still feel close to them." Karol and I began considering how we could design a diverse series of personal grief rituals to strengthen continuing bonds, each of which could be molded to the unique relationship she enjoyed with her father, her two colleagues, and Samantha. Perhaps she could write journaling entries to her colleagues or put aside time to talk with her father? But Karol had already been consumed by a perpetual loop of past dialogues that reverberated through her mind; she was adrift and detached from the conversations playing out in front of her. Might it be good to embody the behaviors of those she lost so as to identify and feel close to them? Perhaps not. Karol spent the previous year cooking familiar meals her colleague had shared with her long ago; dinnertime with her family left her chewing food in silence, staring miles beyond the table and imagining what

DOI: 10.4324/9781351204873-7

her friend Samantha would have been able to still eat at the end of her life while in hospice. It was increasingly apparent to both Karol and me that she was drowning in reverie, engulfed in the past at the expense of a neglected present. I suggested that she may, in fact, benefit from being *less* connected to her losses. Karol's breath quivered in a sudden and dramatic inhale. Her eyes widened. Her body jerked away from me ever so slightly, as if I were brandishing a knife. Every fiber of her being shook with panic as she exhaled a deep breath of air she had been holding a few seconds too long. Karol turned her gaze up and inward towards her mind, as if hoping to find that her father, her two beloved colleagues, and Samantha were all still there.

The tenacious and dogged wisdom of moving on

After all that death has destroyed and left shattered on the ground, beyond the heartache of picking up every broken shard of a war-torn and weary heart, a future pregnant with life beats beneath the rubble, waiting to be built back up and born anew. The bereaved must, in due time, orient themselves once more to a life filled with meaning and joy. To reconstruct one's life following the death of a loved one undoubtedly demands Herculean grit and resolve. Great energy must be summoned to adapt and move forward, but from what reserves? It seems that those faculties previously devoted to relinquishing what came before are to be redirected towards embracing all that life still has to offer. Nonetheless, we are left to wonder: At what point in time should energy be withdrawn from the past and devoted to life after a loss?

Rituals and various customs around the world have a built-in, definitive end point at which time formal mourning behaviors are to be drawn to a close. Subsequent to their cessation, the bereaved are ushered back into life according to cultural values that dictate the precise parameters for when grief is and is no longer appropriate. Some are strikingly succinct. Taoists typically mourn for a period of forty-nine days (Crowder, 2003). Traditional Hindu practices devote the thirteen days following a death for family members to grieve (Cush et al., 2008). Muslims may only afford the bereaved three days (Yasien-Esmael & Rubin, 2005). The Ojibwe tribe of North America hold a four-day wake during which surviving tribespeople say goodbye to the deceased; its brevity encourages a return to normal life soon after a loss (Walker-Gillet, 2011).

Other cultures extend mourning over notably longer stretches of time. In the Philippines, the soul of the deceased is believed to wander for forty days. Wakes and vigils are held for the dead, and a special prayer is read aloud on the fortieth day to help the soul ascend to the afterlife. For the bereaved, however, life grinds to a screeching halt. It is customary in Filipino culture to wear a black pin or adorn oneself completely in black clothing for the entire first year after a death. Family members refrain from celebrations, and widows are barred from remarrying or removing their wedding rings. This moratorium on life finally lifts during *babang luksa*. Translated as *lowering of mourning*, this ritual marks the end of formal mourning exactly one year following the death. Family members of the deceased are permitted to resume wearing colored clothing and may once again host birthday celebrations and attend parties; the spouse of the deceased is also permitted to remarry should he or she choose to do so (Santiago, 1993).

But not all cultures adhere to a fixed allotment of days. The conclusion of mourning may be more contingent upon certain events that unfold at a variable pace. The Japanese practice of ancestor worship regularly spans decades and reaches across numerous generations. Mourning for the deceased ancestor is thought to continue unabated until every surviving family member who ever walked alongside the deceased no longer treads upon the terrain of this world (Hori, 1994).

Some peoples' customs task the bereaved to wait patiently and persist in mourning over many years while the deceased's remains slowly rot. The Choctaw Native Americans of Oklahoma once practiced a *double burial*, a second and more resolute interment of the deceased's bones. After being picked clean of what flesh still clung to the bone, the dry remains were buried beneath a mound of earth and stones and no longer brought out for tribal gatherings, marking a definitive transition beyond mourning (Kidwell, 2007). The Malagasy of Madagascar still practice *famadihana*, with its prolonged liminal phase of mourning in which the deceased are not considered truly dead until the body has decayed in full. Following an initial burial, the body is exhumed every five to seven years for ceremonial dancing and conversation until its complete decomposition is confirmed; only then are death and the mourning process considered complete (Holloway, 2014).

Whether mourning and its rituals are to last three days or span three generations, most cultures believe that a myopic focus on the past must open once more to take in a lively existence grounded in the here and now. The ritual must end. This collective wisdom jibes well with insights regarding psychological health after a loss. Mourning that continues in perpetuity gives way to chronic malady. Uninterrupted engagement in grief rituals can degenerate over time into compulsive routines that sustain adhesion to the past. Consider the bereaved individual who visits the grave site of a loved one every Saturday. This ritualized behavior may have once been a meaningful act that helped confront the reality of a loss, that induced healthy expressions of sorrow, or provided circumscribed time to feel connected to the dead, but the ritual no longer proves beneficial if done merely out of rote habit or if it functions as a fearful evasion of future developments.

Much of the mourning process finds one naturally oriented towards the deceased's departure from this world. The bereaved shed tears over their absence, bid them farewell, and negotiate abstract ties that reach out to the dead from where the living still stand. But overwhelming consensus among psychologists warrants forward movement as a marker of healthy mourning.

It is imperative that the bereaved eventually point their feet towards what lies ahead. In each individual's own way, they must transcend beyond their previous life and arrive at a new plane of existence without the deceased's external presence.

William Worden's task model asserts that one of four major components of mourning entails *adjusting to a world without the deceased*. Therese Rando's six-R process charges the bereaved to *readjust to the world* after a death and move forward *without forgetting*. The dual process model of coping with bereavement (DPM) insists that it is crucial to oscillate back and forth between the *loss-oriented* stresses of relinquishing a relationship and the *restoration-oriented* stresses of managing life as it moves ahead.

A host of cultural grief rituals seems to intuit this seesaw balancing act: An occasional return to grief and remembrance can embolden the living and propel them forward. Tradition may proclaim that a bereft community is to be pulled out of mourning in due time and thrust back into life, but the bereaved are buoyed by the promise of revisiting delimited acts of memorialization at fixed moments ahead. Commenting on the Ojibwe, Walker-Gillet (2011) states, "Each year, at a designated time, the community holds a feast to remember those who have died throughout the past year. Death is accepted as a Rite of Passage into the next phase of the soul's journey" (p. 99). It is customary for Hindus to draw formal mourning to a close thirteen days after a death, only to return for monthly and annual *sraddhas* that set aside momentary breaks from day-to-day life to grieve and encourage the deceased's soul to join all other ancestors in the afterlife (Cush et al., 2008). And in Japan, perennial reliance upon ancestor worship brackets off time every year for the living to step away from their busy lives to invite the dead back into the home.

The Jewish ritual of reciting Kaddish, often referred to as *the mourner's prayer*, is infused with multiple layers of meaning. Children of the deceased are expected to quote the prayer verbatim every Sabbath service for eleven months after a loss, and the entire family partakes in its reading on the anniversary of the loved one's death. By participating in this ritual, those in mourning remain close in spirit to the deceased. But Kaddish also marks an important transition into the future. Mourning beyond the first year is generally discouraged, as it is believed that surviving family members should be fully integrated back into normal life and no longer consumed with grief (Levine, 1997). And yet during every anniversary of the death, the entire congregation joins family members of the deceased as they once more recite Kaddish, an ephemeral moment to summon memories of the deceased before returning again to a life the dead no longer inhabit.

Culture heartens its bereaved community with a predictable timetable for both the expression of grief and the eventual cessation of mourning, but the individual may find that the number of allotted days is awkwardly imposed, concluding too abruptly or dragging on for too long. And insofar as cultural traditions provide a roadmap for *how* to move forward after a loss, the prescribed path may not guide one towards where they most need to travel. In such instances, the individual can deploy personal grief rituals that determine when, according to one's preferred pace, mourning will truly come to an end.

Personal grief rituals can also mark transitions into new territory by means of one's desired route, be it a relinquishing of old symbols or an embrace of something entirely unrelated to previous attachments. Reeves (2011) observed the value of ritual symbols that pertain to past and present experiences of loss, but also those that represent future-oriented hopes and dreams that rise from the ashes of mourning. The bereaved can carve out time for novel activities, to nurture new relationships, or to incorporate symbols that represent growth and an ecstatic thirst for life – all while still affording opportunity to take respite from future developments and revisit the past as needed. These expressions of mourning will be particularly helpful for those whose attachment to the deceased has left them chained to loss-oriented stress about the deceased's time on earth in neglect of what remains of their own.

The attachment perspective: Should I stay behind, or should I go ahead?

The human animal is painfully ambivalent about growth. A child makes herself breakfast for the first time without her father's assistance and quietly yearns for the dependence that no longer defines their bond. A young man writes a paper for school without consulting his mother, whose guidance he relied upon for so long, and feels a twinge of loneliness swell in his chest as he completes his assignment unassisted. Margaret Mahler (1972), a developmental psychologist, once stated, "Inherent in every new step of independent functioning is a minimal threat of object loss." (p. 333). Indeed, she argued that psychological development invariably moves us away from our most intense attachments, thus representing a lifelong process of mourning. But the child does not walk towards autonomy in a straight line. Just as emerging independence piques separation anxiety and motivates the occasional trip back home, so too does adaptation to loss and grief motivate a return to some approximation of ongoing connection to the deceased attachment figure. Perhaps this is why so many cultural rituals and traditions carry an implicit message that mourning, though it may be drawn to a close, can be opened up again. A community steeped in its progression beyond the past will regularly circle back to grieve, remember the relationships they have lost along the way, and feel the deceased's presence for a moment, only to hurry ahead once more to resume forward movement. Each bereaved individual within a community of many must negotiate their desire to voyage ahead with the discomfort of moving further away from one's most cherished attachments. How can this be managed?

Mahler's observations on psychological development provide commentary on how young children learn to navigate the challenges of separation alongside the drive towards independence. During the rapprochement crisis, there is a back-and-forth toggling between closeness and distance, along with their associated points of anxiety: enmeshment and utter abandonment. The child, who may find his mother's constant embrace to be rather suffocating, is enthused to set out into an uncharted world beyond the familiarity of her lap but soon finds the journey has brought him further away than he can tolerate, prompting a panicked retreat to his secure base to ensure mother is still there to hold him. Over time, the little girl or boy will hopefully develop *object constancy*, an internalized representation of the attachment figure's presence. Fortified with trust that the caregiver remains available even when out of sight, the child feels comfortable enough to continue their courageous exploration of the world away from home.

Mahler's theory of *separation-individuation* jibes quite well with the DPM and its prescription for how to best cope with bereavement. Ideally, one can oscillate between mediations on the past and engagement with the present. They can stay near to recollections of the deceased at times and, at other moments, step away from memory to tackle new tasks and form new bonds. She seeks out the internal mental representation of the dead, conjures up the past, and actively grieves what has been lost (loss-oriented stress). She then reorients her mind towards the stress of all that awaits as her life continues to unfold (restoration-oriented stress).

This balancing act is all possible because of secure attachment and the achievement of object constancy. The bereaved individual is better able to engage in life without the dead if they trust that continuing bonds are available as needed. Repeated confrontations with both types of stress yield confidence that neither will negate the other: grief work need not obstruct further growth, nor will the pursuit of life after a loss render reflections on the past inaccessible. I use the phrase *absence-and-presence* to denote this capacity to move through a world in which the deceased's absence is acknowledged while also maintaining access to the deceased's enduring presence within the mind.

But for those saddled with insecure attachment and a lack of object constancy, making room for grief and forward movement is a zero-sum game. Oscillations do not occur because one side of the equation is approached in excess while the other is neglected. Some are too eager to abandon ties to the past; they run towards what is next with the enthusiasm of a child releasing mother's hand to explore a new playground. This is particularly the case for those with a dismissing attachment style who have seemed to deactivate thoughts about the attachment figure. A dearth of object constancy is apparent when the internal representation of the deceased is either not sought out for comfort or lacks an emotional connotation when memory is cued. They may appear to be getting on with their lives untethered to what came before, but the outright avoidance of efforts to cope with loss-oriented stress can rear its head in unconscious compulsions to maintain negative continuing bonds or inadvertent self-sabotage of the very growth and development they claim to be after. Personal grief rituals that facilitate forward movement are contraindicated when the bereaved is already moving ahead too quickly. These individuals would be better served by ritualized activities that confirm true acceptance of loss and absence (see Chapter 4), magnify emotional expression (see Chapter 5), or carve out room for continuing bonds (see Chapter 6).

Others cling too tight to mourning. Memories about the deceased and the outpourings of grief they stir up, though painful, are subjectively experienced as a treasured connection to the deceased. To move forward in time is felt to be tantamount to leaving the dead behind, forever out of reach, and so the individual may hesitate to relinquish their grip on the past and walk into a world the dead never knew. When preoccupied attachment style is at play, the course of mourning is often characterized by heightened affective display of pain and excessive access to memories of the deceased that only perpetuate emotional distress. The preoccupied individual does not trust that the memory of the deceased will remain available and intact should they branch out for a while away from their familiar home. Furthermore, they are encumbered by an internal working model that doubts their own ability to maneuver through life. And so they inhibit exploration of what lies ahead and opt to stay put, preferring to vigilantly monitor the internal presence of those strong figures they always relied upon to allay their fears.

For these individuals, ever-present continuing bonds and unrelenting grief saturate the ground beneath their feet, hindering forward movement like so much quicksand. They would be aided by personal grief rituals that lift them out of perpetual mourning and partition time and space to tackle the challenges of life without the deceased and experience life anew. The challenge often lies in judiciously removing those cues that summon excessive reminders of the past without making rash attempts to goad them into moving on, which would only trigger panic about memories eroding and any semblance of a meaningful tie fading away. Continuing bonds must be compartmentalized with the promise of being able to return. Anything short of this would be commensurate with asking a child to abruptly leave home and instantaneously grow forever calm and confident in their independence, no longer in need of homecoming.

Let us now return to the case of Karol and how she was able to overcome her crippling fear that she would lose access to memories of those she loved and lost. Karol struggled to engage with life as it marched forward in front of her eyes. And our original efforts to increase continuing bonds would have only fixed her gaze further on what was no longer there. We soon endeavored to design a personal grief ritual that could help her be more absorbed in the here and now while trusting that she could resume contemplating the past as needed. She and I sustained our focus on this dilemma. In the middle of one such therapy session, Karol spontaneously blurted out, "I could make a memory box!" She explained that it might help to use small pieces of paper to jot down fond memories of time spent with friends and family she had lost, including simple notes about their more pronounced attributes and how each person impacted her life. She wanted to place these folded pieces of paper into individual matchboxes with the deceased's name written on them. I shared my understanding that storing these memories somewhere safe would give her the peace of mind she needed to focus more on her present-day life, free from concerns of amnesia.

Karol arrived at my office the following week clutching a weathered wooden keepsake box she had retrieved from the back corner of a storage unit. Much of the dark walnut finish had been chipped away; its gold trim had clearly lost its original brilliance. The rusty hinges creaked as Karol opened the lid to reveal its contents: a mound of blank pieces of paper and an assortment of empty matchboxes waiting to be filled with tiny reminiscences. She began one appointment after the next by withdrawing a scrap of paper, elaborating on a fond memory she wished to hold on to, and writing a summary of what had been at the forefront of her mind for so many years. I merely provided an audience for Karol's nostalgia. She harked back to echoes of her childhood and the words of wisdom her father imparted her way before his mental faculties eluded him. One session was devoted towards recalling funny moments from a trip she and a colleague had taken to Italy. A few larger pieces of paper detailed some of her favorite recipes for homemade bread and lasagna that her colleague had passed along.

And then there was Samantha, who had accompanied Karol through their mutual ordeal with breast cancer. Karol jotted down various memories of how their budding friendship began and grew stronger even as Samantha succumbed to relapse many years after Karol had recovered. She encased each of these recollections into a separate matchbox with the person's name written on the outside before placing it into the wooden box with the rest. Following numerous enactments of this personal grief ritual, Karol was breathing with greater ease. Most noticeably, I will never forget how her gaze softened as she said, "Now I know they're there if I need them."

Karol's unique use of the memory box she created eased her concerns about forgetting the past. And she maintained conscious acknowledgment of the ritual's meaning, that the matchboxes represented memories of past relationships she had permanently lost, memories she no longer needed to anxiously monitor. This proved to be a healthy act of mourning, as evidenced by Karol becoming more engaged with her closest relationships in the here and now. Despite her dread, she was better able to trust that she could return when needed to the old, weathered box and the scraps of nostalgia they harbored within.

Two steps forward, one step back: The many causes for ambivalence when adapting to loss

The bereaved may bemoan the burden of shouldering sorrow, and yet many of his behaviors reveal marked ambivalence about lightening the load. A deep schism lies between the acute pains of grief and the life that awaits on the other side. Those with a preoccupied attachment style *are* more prone to a chronic course of grief and mourning. But regardless of one's interpersonal proclivities, the prospect of investing energy into surviving relationships or creating something new after a loss is fraught with conflict and mixed feelings for many. The past tempts those in mourning to linger, like a friend enticing you to stay for one more libation even though your feet are pointing towards the door. Psychological factors that motivate one to remain stalled are plentiful, often lurking undetected within the mind. If personal grief rituals are to assist the bereaved in adapting to life after a loss, the meaning behind each individual's reluctance to move forward must be coaxed out and considered with empathy at the outset of a ritual's design.

Many of these inhibitions are tied to an overarching theme of separation anxiety. *The passing of time* in and of itself is enough to foster such fear. As if one were literally drifting farther away from a loved one, the ever-widening gap between the last moment of interaction with the deceased and the present moment is subjectively experienced as an increasingly unbearable distance. With no control over the clock, the bereaved reach back in time and cling with desperation to what fleeting reminiscences remain. Grief, with its perseveration of thoughts about the deceased and persistent yearning for proximity to the deceased, becomes the last bastion of attachment. The more ideal solution, of course, is to maintain healthy continuing bonds with the dead that provide meaningful connection while also paving a path upon which new life can be explored. But uncharted ground can be frightening, and so the bereaved brood over loss-oriented nostalgia and hitch themselves to the familiar, albeit debilitating pain of grief.

Or it may be that the future is avoided for *fear of forgetting the past*. Musings on the past can soothe what aches, but they are susceptible to decay over time. New experiences may come to be seen as the coup de grâce that renders the dead forever irretrievable, a clanging cacophony of fresh memories that drown out fading echoes of old. Such was Karol's concern as she anxiously monitored the internal presence of those she had lost. The past is preserved at the expense of a neglected present, like a concertgoer who fails to enjoy one note of music because she is too bent on capturing a photograph of each ephemeral moment.

The threat of forward movement and adaptation may even lie in a fear that *change will render the bereaved unrecognizable and incapable of being found!* In mourning, the attachment system remains equipped with an impulse to beckon attachment figures nearer in hopes that the dead will step out of the void to seek reunion. Mummification, the instinct to preserve rooms and inanimate objects exactly as they were before death arrived, is often fueled by an unconscious fantasy that the dead just might return, but only if they are welcomed back into familiar surrounds. The same instinct may be applied towards preservation of the self. Some are beset with a quiet fear that, should they change, the deceased will return only to find that they do not recognize who the bereaved has become. A client of mine once expressed a great degree of unease after getting a new haircut, stating that her deceased friend "wouldn't even know me if he saw me now." The bereaved might attempt to quell separation anxiety by halting change and growth, standing still, and waiting for the dead to find them just as they were before.

In AD 79, as the city of Pompeii was suffocating beneath volcanic ash and rubble, Pliny the Younger watched from afar as the fiery chaos consumed nearly 2,000 souls, including his uncle. While recounting the ordeal to a friend, Pliny the Younger (1963) wrote:

> I could boast that not a groan or cry of fear escaped me in those perils, but I admit that I derived some poor consolation in my mortal lot from the belief that the whole world was dying with me and I with it.
>
> (p. 166)

Such honest introspection about his experience of surviving death highlights just how beguiling it can be to stay connected to the dead rather than pick up the pieces, separate from past ties, and carry on without them. For those who fail to resist this pull, there ensues a symbolic death of the self, a cessation of growth as payment for an eternal link to the deceased attachment figure. They may even opt to sidestep any potential joys or meaningful bonds that lie ahead for fear that those, too, will be buried under the unforgiving weight of time and mortality and force another trial of separation, what Otto Rank (1945) once described as *life fear*.

An entirely different source of conflict centers on moralistic anxieties. Some bereaved individuals wrestle with a belief, however irrational, that adapting to life after a loss amounts to some wrongdoing on their part. Being at odds with one's conscience is cause for clinical concern, as prolonged guilt can derail efforts to cope with the stress of living in the wake of mourning (Prigerson & Jacobs, 2001; Stroebe et al., 2014). And the bereaved may hesitate to engage in rituals that take on future-oriented stresses and joys if they harbor self-critical attitudes about moving forward.

One such challenge to healthy bereavement comes in the form of what William Worden (2008) called *recovery guilt*, a belief that the memory of the deceased has been dishonored should the bereaved "move through grief and want to get on with their lives" (pg. 225). This concern may very well be rooted in childhood anxieties about abandoning mother or father if ever one grows up and moves away, a curious reversal of separation anxiety dynamics (Weiss, 1993). Following a loss, filling the void with new relationships or activities may be seen as an act of betrayal, a retroactive devaluation of what came before as something easily replaceable. Simply *being able to adjust to life without the deceased*, the bereaved worries, can be viewed as commensurate with an insignificant attachment that had not been especially important;

the bereaved may then come to find virtue in remaining stuck in chronic grief as an homage to the deceased. Thus, much of recovery guilt stems from an erroneous conviction that the bereaved must choose between being fully committed to past memories or disrespectfully leaving the dead and their legacy behind.

Recovery guilt is made exponentially worse by concerns that family, friends, and members of the community will cast stones should the individual improve. Chronic mourning may then be motivated less by authentic pangs of grief, serving instead as a disingenuous show of misery that broadcasts what is assumed to be an appropriate response to loss. These assumptions about others' judgments may very well be a projection of one's own moral strictures. Either way, the rigid and unforgiving thought processes that fuel recovery guilt must be examined and extinguished before enacting personal grief rituals that center on new activities or new relationships.

The sheer presence of anything new after a loss may be enough to spark concerns that something is morally amiss. But mourning abhors a vacuum. The death of an attachment figure leaves an absence that pulls for potential replacements in order to heal. Time once spent with the dying can now be devoted to other meaningful activities. Intimacy and connection reserved for those no longer alive can be used to strengthen surviving ties. And much of what fills the vacuum emerges in a nascent state brimming with potential, born out of the ashes of what has been lost: motivation to build a new career, to foster a new romantic relationship, or to cultivate more mature outlook on the futility of stressing trivial problems. Death may even deliver tangibles to the bereaved, such as real estate, an inheritance, or valued family heirlooms. Loss, it seems, begets gains.

This sequence of death giving way to new life is, for some, misconstrued as something to feel self-conscious about, as if embracing what follows loss is tantamount to *having willingly agreed to an objectionable trade: In exchange for new life, I welcome the other's death.* To benefit from loss is taken to be a deal with the devil that stokes eternal guilt and self-punishment, often manifesting as inhibition about growth and forward movement. Some examples are rather straightforward, such as a relative of the deceased who uses an inheritance to buy a new home for their family only to feel sullen and undeserving upon moving in. But the subjective sense that one has made an amoral trade can find obscure routes of expression. Jennifer, whose loss of her thirty-six-year-old son from lung cancer was discussed in Chapter 5, was gripped by disquieting anxiety upon becoming a grandmother after her surviving son had his first child. We soon discovered that she was bearing an implicit thought that, by enjoying time with her growing family, one life had been willingly sacrificed for the other.

Lastly, the bereaved may feel uneasy about *outliving the dead and partaking in what the deceased never got to experience.* Continuing to thrive after the deceased has departed can be seen as a competition which survivors have mixed feelings about winning, as if they were greedily gobbling up a present moment without consideration for the deceased person's hunger for more life. This particular experience of guilt about adapting to life without the deceased can be rather insidious. It deserves an in-depth analysis, and in doing so we now turn to the psychoanalyst Melanie Klein (1940) and her conceptualization of *triumph* as it relates to complicated mourning.

Klein begins with the observation that, from infancy through old age, dependence on others inspires great ambivalence. Yes, mutual attachment provides emotional security, but behaviors designed to maintain proximity to mother and father are rooted in the basic presupposition that we are weak in isolation and lacking in some essential way. The realization that we require others to function most optimally is not only a blow to our confidence and sense of self-efficacy, but dependency also puts us in a precarious position, always at risk of catastrophe should we lose our relationships.

Klein astutely observed that some people attempt to deny a detestable sense of dependency by contemptuously devaluing what the attachment figure has to offer, subsequently viewing oneself as fully self-sufficient. The other is not only seen as having nothing of value that does not already reside within the self, but their absence is also regarded as inconsequential, even a welcome departure. This is Klein's notion of *triumph*, a reversing of the polarities regarding who within a dyad is big and who is small, who is strong and who is weak.

Klein's theories were sensitive to the thin veil between a confident grasp on external reality and the subjective experience that one's internal mediations have real consequences. She posited that the mere fantasy of trivializing and disparaging a relationship, ultimately an aggressive wish that it be destroyed, yields to concerns that the fantasy has caused legitimate harm to the much-needed attachment figure. When death actually rips the other away, subsequent mourning can stoke intense guilt about unconscious wishes for triumph having contributed to the deceased's demise. Anger, once directed towards dependence upon the relationship in a bid for strength and independence, is now directed towards the self as punishment for having ever wished to surpass the other.

Betty, a single woman in her sixties, sought out grief therapy with me shortly after slogging her way back to Chicago from her father's funeral in upstate Maine. We met for a few appointments in my office, but she soon made it clear that the real work needed to take place within her home. Betty held out her phone to show me pictures of the cluttered mess in her walk-up apartment that I would become accustomed to stepping around for the next three years: boxes spilling over with unopened mail, rusted cookware strewn about the kitchen countertops, an uninviting arrangement of furniture piled high with old coats, and heaps of dusty books crammed into rickety shelves.

Of greatest significancc was the collection of computers and numerous components acquired over three decades that now littered the floor. There were word processors, extracted motherboards and hard drives, stacks of floppy disks, personal computers, plastic bins filled with power cords and miscellaneous wires, external speakers, keyboards, mouses and mouse pads, modems, monitors, and various laptops. I was not surprised to find that this jumble of relics had meaningful ties to her relationship with her father; each outmoded technology still carried memories of him stopping by to string together a mess of wires for her and assemble the newest device she had purchased. I was caught off guard, however, by her subjective experience of what she needed most in order to mourn his absence. Betty did not mind the clutter at all, as was apparent after a year of half-hearted attempts to discard anachronistic junk from her home. She was, in fact, more weighed down by guilt about wanting to buy yet another computer: a touchscreen tablet. She revealed that doing so would be the first piece of new technology acquired since her father passed. Betty felt ill at ease about this prospect, not only because she would be experiencing some aspect of life he never got to hold in his hands, but also because this would be the first time for her setting up a novel device without needing her father's assistance.

Betty ended up purchasing the tablet despite her moralistic qualms. We put aside time for her to open the box and set up her new toy, thus enacting newfound independence and forward movement into a future of technologies her father would never have been able to imagine. I asked her what she was feeling as she connected each cord in its rightful place. With shaky hands and tearful eyes, she said, "I feel like I'm in trouble, like I'm doing something wrong, like I'm killing Dad." Betty and I sat still amid the chaotic sprawl. We learned to leave the old clothes, books, and electronics undisturbed and focused our conversations instead on the opportunities she still had to strike out into the future and bring new life into her home.

Presence of the present moment: Rituals that fill the void of absence with something new

Most bereaved individuals manage to embrace the paradox of absence-and-presence: They let go of past ties while simultaneously maintaining an approximation of continuing bonds. Personal grief rituals assist in negotiating this balancing act, confronting the reality of loss vis-à-vis an illusory presence of the very person whose absence is being mourned. Memories are rekindled through storytelling. Old haunts are visited and experienced as portals to what the relationship once felt like. Imaginary conversations with the dead entail observations of their passing. But must all grief rituals be devoted to what came before?

Healthy mourning entails the felt presence of a past relationship as well as the presence of new life in the here and now. Both play complementary roles in filling the void of absence. The fresh sounds of conversation with the living and novel experiences vibrate in harmony with echoes of the past. In those instances when the bereaved would benefit from stronger footing in the present moment, personal grief rituals can impel them to seek out new relationships, reside in unfamiliar spaces, and create new memories through unusual activities.

Enacting new activities

Jocelyn, whose efforts to confront her father's absence at the workbench in the garage were discussed in Chapter 4, continued to live at home with her mother. The house required ongoing maintenance, and without their family's patriarch there to make repairs, Jocelyn stood in his stead. She rewired the ceiling fan when it stopped revolving. She built her mother a step stool to use in the kitchen when reaching for cookware stored on the highest shelves. She installed insulation in the attic before the winter arrived. Jocelyn enjoyed this hands-on approach to mourning. But the persistent pain of grief still left her wondering what else she could do to cope.

A year after her loss, Jocelyn considered taking a woodworking class to learn more about what she wished her father had been able to teach her. We discussed how this might be a meaningful way to mourn: She would still be able to acknowledge her father's absence while, at the same time, maintaining continuing bonds by incorporating more of his behaviors. But Jocelyn never took the class. Week after week, she forgot to register, or she would work extra shifts at her job that conflicted with the class schedule. I offered an interpretation: Despite her initial excitement, perhaps she had mixed feelings about taking on *more* activities that would provoke thoughts about her father. Jocelyn, in her characteristically dry manner, simply nodded and said, "Yep." She and I were both surprised by the intense aggravation in her voice as she exclaimed, "I'm *always* thinking about my dad. If I'm not doing things he used to do, or things we used to do together, I'm talking to someone about him or sharing memories with my family about him." A constant barrage of her father's presence, in both memory and action, had consumed her life. The past encroached upon her space, smothering each attempt to breathe in the present moment.

Jocelyn's case exemplifies how remaining engaged in activities once done with the deceased, discussing the dead with others, or taking on behaviors they once performed can leave one mired in stale remains of old. Under the guise of continuing bonds or pragmatic efforts to fill vacant roles in the family and community, excessive loss-oriented stress can contribute to a chronic course of grief. Preoccupied and exhausted from unremitting reminiscence, the bereaved may fare better pursuing activities with no meaningful tie to the deceased.

Though Jocelyn wished that her father could still be standing by her at the workbench, she yearned to break free from the space he occupied in her mind. With each twist of a wire between her fingers and each torque of a wrench, every movement left her feeling as if she did not know where her father's life ended and where hers began. We started to discuss how she could set aside time for a recurring personal grief ritual in which she would do something entirely different from anything she and her father ever did together. She was eager to begin. However, their lives and interests had been so intertwined that Jocelyn struggled to think of what would afford her separation. We spent the next two appointments brainstorming and mulling over a short list of novel activities she could incorporate into a personal grief ritual.

Jocelyn was soon regaling me with stories of ventures that felt radically foreign and, at the same time, quite refreshing. She and her friends did a Segway tour of downtown Chicago. She took knife-throwing classes, which found her methodically flinging large blades at old wooden planks set up in nearby alleyways. Lastly, Jocelyn proclaimed that she wanted to dress differently. She and her father, ever the kindred spirits, even dressed in similar wardrobes cut from the same cloth. Every hooded sweatshirt and pair of faded blue jeans she wore further evoked her father's presence when she looked in the mirror. And so she set aside time to augment her attire. More than mere shopping sprees, excursions into unfamiliar clothing stores and boutiques came to represent meaningful departures from a past that had grown threadbare. She began wearing stylish leggings and linen pants, sundresses and jumpsuits, turtlenecks, and cardigan sweaters. And still, hoodies and jeans maintained a regular place in her rotation of outfits. One of my last memories of Jocelyn is of her sitting in my office, recounting how she had recently caught a glimpse of herself reflected in a pane of glass in one of the alleyways where she and her new friends met to practice their knife-throwing skills. The woman she saw was pitching sharp blades at plywood targets with impressive accuracy, all while donning a new leather jacket. And though her evolved sense of self brought a smirk upon her face, she wished her father could see her transformation for himself.

Nurturing new relationships

John Bowlby (1963) observed that it is commonplace for the bereaved to cope with loss by assuming roles left unfilled after the deceased's passing. A sociodynamic perspective helps us understand how this is an adaptive response to loss, particularly for the well-being of a reeling community. Bowlby stated, "In every social group roles are distributed asymmetrically among individuals so that, when one is removed, disequilibrium results. In such circumstances there is pressure on one or other of those remaining to assume the role of the absentee" (p. 516).

In addition to the reassignment of roles, relationships may also be rearranged after a death. The LoDagaa of West Africa hold numerous ceremonies in the months that follow a loss to help members of their community transition into vacant roles and responsibilities, claim possessions, and reorganize themselves into new friendships and romantic partnership. Though the deceased is still being slowly relinquished, not yet entirely absent from the community members' hearts and minds, society moves forward nonetheless during this liminal phase of mourning and adaptation (Goody, 1962).

The bereaved individual often benefits from a liminal process of slow separation from the dead alongside the emerging development of new relationships. This is apparent in the friendships Jocelyn formed while she gradually teased apart the tight bond she had with her father. Personal grief rituals can be designed to encourage the pursuit and nurturance of novel attachments in the here and now. But the relational wheel need not be reinvented. Relationships that already exist can be folded into pre-existing means of connection. Those meaningful activities once associated with a unique tie to the departed can be played out with surviving members of the community, friends, and family members *of the individual's choosing*. This reassigning of roles is quite adaptive throughout mourning insofar as the new relationship does not amount to a simple *substitute* that merely supplants the deceased and glosses over the pain of loss as if a loved one never died.

Recall Libby from the previous chapter, who used personal grief rituals to remain connected to her mother as she traveled to cities and tourist sites around the world. As discussed, she also sought out familiar bike paths and bookstores they used to frequent together, all with a sense that her mother was right there with her. Each of these activities uplifted her as she continued to mourn. Nonetheless, her mother's absence still weighed heavy, and Libby felt lonely. It no longer felt sufficient to summon an illusory sense of her mother's nearness while working on household projects; she wanted someone to actually help her steady a frame she was hanging. She grew tired of imagining that her mother was beside her as she wrapped Christmas presents; she hoped to invite someone else to keep her company – one of her young daughters, perhaps. Libby started to suspect that a different kind of personal grief ritual was necessary to quell the pains of absence, one that would incorporate a new relationship into her old routines.

Libby was readying herself and her children to embark on a road trip with her husband's family, and the driving arrangements had Libby paired with only her mother-in-law. Though they had always gotten along perfectly well, they never seemed to have much to discuss beyond basic pleasantries and small talk. Plus, the trip was estimated to last eighteen hours! She worried about how they would pass the time, which brought to mind memories of listening to audiobooks whenever she and her mother were stuck in the car for a long jaunt. Libby felt sad as she reminisced about the simple joy of basking in storytelling and then talking with her mother about what they had just taken in. She had long been perturbed about how, following her mother's death, there were few surviving family members with whom she could discuss books. The one exception was her mother-in-law, who was also an avid reader, albeit of wildly different genres and tastes.

Libby planned to ask her in advance about a book or two that they might both appreciate. Libby proposed one that was more her style – she enjoyed nonfiction accounts of history – and also invited her mother-in-law, who favored fictional detective stories, to suggest one of her liking. The ritual, if you will, was the intentional initiation of her listening to audiobooks with someone new. Though she fretted at first that her mother-in-law would abhor the experience or that they would have nothing to say to each other, Libby was overjoyed to find that the conversation flowed with ease. It was bitter-sweet to evoke a reminder of her mother's absence, but this personal grief ritual helped Libby forge a deeper bond with a surviving family member while simultaneously reawakening a cherished pastime she feared she would never be able to share with anyone again.

Opening new space in the home

Home is the nexus of one's most significant relationships, where family and friends gather to deepen their bonds. It is quite fitting, then, that the home-stead provides the central location wherein many cultures choose to mourn their dead. Some peoples summon the community into their abode to con-front the deceased's absence and express grief; notable practices include those of Hawaiians, the Ifugao people of the Philippines, and the Jewish ritual of sitting shiva. And various domiciles around the world house acts of continu-ing bonds with the dead, including the Torajans of Indonesia and the practice of ancestor worship in Japan.

Other rituals demarcate space within the home to nurture new experiences and relationships. The front door often serves as the most powerful symbol, a partition between death that has been buried beneath the ground and left outside . . . and all that is blooming with vitality and potential inside. Crow-der (2003), remarking about the Chinese, observed, "Funeral guests make a detour on the way home to leave the death airs elsewhere" (pg. 681). The Zulu people of South Africa make sure to wash off any dirt from the burial still clinging to their clothes and skin before walking through the front door (Kotze et al., 2012).

While these and other cultural rituals emphasize the need to keep death and excessive grief *out* of the home, bereaved individuals intuitively understand the complementary value of actively inviting life back *in*. Thus, one's home becomes a metaphor for healthy mourning: a balancing act of relinquishing enough of the past so as to make room for the present moment. Personal grief rituals carried out within the home can focus on the important task of clearing away an overabundance of links to what is old and stale just as much as they can usher in what is fresh and alive. Also, the privacy inherent within a place of residence may make it a preferable location for authentic and meaningful acts of mourning, as opposed to public burial sites or places of worship that pressure the individual to grieve in a manner that meets others' expectations.

Betty managed to remove some clutter from her apartment, including an assortment of old electronic materials that were obstructing her ability to use her desk, but it was the acquisition and use of a new computer within her home that proved to be the most meaningful push against chronic grief. Rick, who used one type of personal grief ritual to let go of his friend Nia, created a different ritual in which he renovated his kitchen and purchased new furniture with the intent purpose of hosting and building new friendships that would breathe fresh air into his domicile. Carina, who sold the house she and her husband lived in for decades, found that the greatest act of mourning was when she moved to a new house and, despite her characteristic shyness, made a concerted effort to open her space to those that would accompany her through retirement.

The cultivation of new experiences after a loss need not supersede those of old entirely. Jocelyn, for instance, retained her lifelong penchant for woodworking even as she pursued a novel interest in knife-throwing. And she continued to wear her tried-and-true hooded sweatshirts and blue jeans in rotation with her new leather jacket. Jocelyn simply added activities through personal grief rituals that augmented her life.

But some acts of mourning represent a separate urge to remove and be done with vestiges of the past. Jocelyn and her father bemoaned their mutual struggles with weight gain and subsequent health problems, some of which disrupted her father's quality of life and ultimately contributed to his demise. Out of concern that she would suffer a similar fate if she held on to this aspect of their relationship, Jocelyn established the exercise regimen and healthy dietary choices that her father long neglected. And with each pound that fell away, so too did a faint trace of their bond.

Like so much dead skin, superfluous ties to the deceased must be shed so that new life can grow. And this is often to the bereaved individual's liking. Though the adhesion to an attachment figure may have been strong, certain aspects of the original bond lose their grip over time. Tattered clothes are discarded. Traditions and hobbies stemming from time spent with the deceased may be abandoned in pursuit of more novel and exciting activities. And illusory conversations with the dead echo less frequently as the bereaved resume their preference for speaking with living souls.

Therein lies the importance of what Van der Hart and Ebbers (1981) called *rites of separation*: Some acts of mourning rouse the bereaved to take leave of the dead and establish symbolic distance from the past. This is why some cultural grief rituals encourage the bereaved to discard or destroy traces of prior attachments. Fire appears to be a common medium. During the Filipino ritual of *babang luksa*, held during the first anniversary of a death to mark the *lowering of mourning*, a large social gathering is held during which nonvaluable belongings are burned to symbolize leaving residue from the past behind (Isidro, 1978). During a typical Chinese funeral, often infused with elements of Taoism and Buddhism, the bereaved are expected to grieve loudly; sorrowful wailing peaks in volume as the eldest son of the deceased nails the coffin shut (Kiong, 1990). Inanimate objects involved in these funerary ceremonies are destroyed or purified immediately afterward to represent separation from a prior state of mourning. The bereaved are then obliged to burn their funerary garb upon returning home. Clothes that the deceased once wore may be burned as well. Approximately seven days after burial, mourning is terminated in a ceremony translated as *putting on the red*, during which white clothes – white traditionally represents death in Chinese culture – are exchanged for those dyed in red, a symbol of good fortune (Watson, 1988).

Some people will always retain a modicum of bittersweet ties to their departed loved ones. Even as they move forward with new relationships into unfamiliar spaces, they hold on to some semblance of their beloved in a spirit of eternal reverence and fond reminiscences. But what of those who wish to do away with the dead altogether? Might ritual be the key that unshackles one from the legacy of a painful relationship and finally gives voice to years of rage and anguish? Can the bereaved create personal grief rituals that purge unhealthy relationships and leave them far behind, forever out of sight?

To take leave of the dead: Using rituals of separation to cast out ghosts

Priscilla readied herself for her husband's funeral, as she was expected to. She donned herself in a black dress complemented by a modest attire of dark hues. Gray gloves. Flat shoes. A simple black hat. Inconspicuous jewelry. A touch of makeup. At the funeral, Priscilla stood still next to her children in a feigned posture of gloom. Family members greeted her with sad expressions and offered their quiet condolences. She nodded and whispered, "Thank you." At the burial site, she politely molded her face into a veil of sorrow, a show of unity with her community of fellow mourners. But when it was time to leave the cemetery, Priscilla let forth a furtive smile she had been biting back all day. Unwilling to express her genuine feelings about the death of her husband, her abuser of over twenty years, she kept a symbol of what his demise meant to *her* concealed throughout the ceremony: red lingerie meant for her and her new partner to enjoy, a personal and deeply meaningful expression of liberation and renewed joy . . . and bitter hatred.

There is immense wisdom in cultural practices that go to great lengths to ensure that the dead do not haunt the living. In the Sanyuan Village of China, kin of the deceased drive away ghosts by wailing and lighting firecrackers immediately after the death. Australian Aboriginals build vast mounds of sticks, dirt, and bark between the graves and their campsites, a partition to protect the village from evil spirits that could otherwise linger and impinge upon new life (McGrath & Phillips, 2008).

Many individuals embroiled in chronic grief do seem haunted by the deceased's looming specter, particularly if the relationship had been a source of constant agony. Their persistent presence festers and reverberates in the mind, perpetuating all that was deleterious to one's psychological health: criticisms, insults, and shame-inspiring doubts. The attachment figure's malevolence seems to jump from its previous host and continue feeding off the survivor's psyche, assailing the bereaved from within.

This subjective phenomenon falls under the category of an *introject*: an internalized mental representation of the other that continues to plague the bereaved from within. Some are tormented more by *linking objects*, those external and inanimate objects unconsciously imbued with the deceased's very essence and related to as stand-ins for their actual presence. In either case, it is imperative to design a personal grief ritual that, like an antibiotic snuffing out an infection, casts out toxic remnants of the dead like the pathogens they are. This approach is decidedly in order if the bereaved thwart their own forward movement after a loss by echoing the deceased's unique brand of discouragement.

Van der Hart and Ebbers (1981) suspected that rites of separation may find their most poignant expression by destroying symbolic objects that represent ties to the dead. But the bereaved must be willing to accept and act on aggressive emotional energy towards memories of the deceased. Furthermore, the underlying meaning of a ritual steeped in feelings of disdain and a desire for distance must be differentiated from similar actions that, say, destroy or get rid of a meaningful symbol for the sake of accepting that a loved one's life has been decimated. Recall the Wari people of Peru, who long practiced endocannibalism. In contrast to the compassion and consideration imbued into the consumption of a deceased community member, devouring the flesh of an enemy slain in battle was carried out with markedly different sentiment. According to Conklin (2007), "Wari see approximately as much similarity between funerary cannibalism and warfare cannibalism as we see between burying our dead and burying our garbage" (p. 1257).

As long as their purpose is clear and the emotional content is tolerated, the benefits of aggressive rites of separation are many. Whatever the method, the bereaved is able to act out their desire for distance from an internal, negative continuing bond. Personal grief rituals that burn fabrics, smash ceramic and glass and metal, or tear paper into ribbons give form to otherwise-amorphous states of hatred and rage. Such violent actions channel fiery emotions felt to be too chaotic to bear internally towards an external symbol that can absorb the attack and show signs of its annihilation. Lastly, obliterating inanimate objects that symbolize an unwelcome presence in the mind may come to feel like a cathartic and overdue clearing of excess debris that had been obstructing the path forward.

One note of caution is in order when enacting this type of personal grief ritual, especially if it hinges upon attempts to exorcise a traumatic relationship.

Judith Herman (1997) was right to note that intrusive memories of abuse and neglect cannot be entirely stamped out and forgotten. It is not advisable to negate the reality of trauma as if it never happened. Instead, memories of such must be integrated alongside a sense of safe distance that allows one to move into a future more decidedly beyond a past riddled with pain.

Priscilla came in for therapy in her fifties. A quick overview of her past revealed that her ex-husband, with whom she had four children, died ten years prior. She did not seem to be struggling with residual feelings of grief, nor were her days colored by a sense of emptiness as a result of his absence. Jay's departure from this world was actually quite welcome, as he had undoubtedly been a malignant force in her life. Priscilla endured merciless critiques and harsh harangues every day over the course of their marriage. The home was never clean enough. Any disruption in the children's behavior was attributed to some shortcoming of hers as a mother. Her career did not generate sufficient income. Struggles with weight gain were not to Jay's liking. Comments at parties they attended fueled angry tirades on the drive home that went on until sunrise, robbing her of any chance to sleep.

Priscilla dreamed of escape. She patiently deliberated over how she and her children could relocate themselves, forever beyond the reach of Jay's unrelenting rage. One day while he was at work, Priscilla sprang into action and absconded with her children to a prearranged refuge at a friend's home, where she proceeded to file for divorce and full custody of the children at a safe distance. Jay died a few years after the divorce was finalized. She went on to form a loving relationship with her new partner in which she explored a sexual renaissance that liberated her, if only partially, from the frustrations of her first marriage. Nonetheless, as Priscilla sat in my office ten years after his death, it was clear that Jay's voice still echoed in the chambers of her mind. The denigrating bond persisted, unabated by his absence.

Priscilla and I spent ample time coaxing out the mixed feelings about Jay's passing she had choked down for decades. Not only had she learned to conceal the slightest tell of her contempt for Jay for fear of stoking his ire, but she also attempted to safeguard her children from the ugliness of their marriage. And as they became adults, she buried the depths of her revulsion behind a facade of humor and minimization. Of greatest concern was that Priscilla often displaced anger and disgust about Jay toward herself. And she did so by mobilizing her familiarity with Jay's malicious style of debasement. An internal dialogue of his caustic tirades stalked her wherever she went. She disparaged herself for every minor mistake she made at work and as a mother. I suggested that her negative feelings about Jay needed to finally be expressed directly at their true target. Priscilla agreed, but she wondered how to level an attack on Jay with him no longer being present to absorb the punches.

During one appointment, Priscilla commented on the vast array of objects still in her house that Jay left behind after the divorce when he was legally required to vacate the family home. Each possession cued distinct recollections of his wrath. The old radio, tucked away in a corner of the basement, still blared reminders of how he played his music loudly with sadistic joy if ever Priscilla tried to rest. Dust-covered cookbooks in the attic sent stale memories floating down into her kitchen from when he would complain about the meals she prepared for him and the children. Priscilla had also held on to his clothes, assuming that her son might need them one day as he grew up. The simple awareness of those shirts and pants in the back of her closet was enough to reawaken Jay's disparaging comments, now experienced as her own self-critical thoughts. I suggested that it was no longer necessary to harbor these things and that she may benefit from finally parting with them. Suddenly, a spark of righteous anger burned in her eyes. She wished to do more than simply relinquish the clutter; she yearned to exorcise her anger and hatred towards something that represented Jay.

Priscilla charted her desired path of destruction. She listed various items that once belonged to Jay and precisely how she would exact years of bottled-up frustration. We discussed how these personal grief rituals could be conducted in private, free from concerns of what others would think of her upset. Priscilla smashed Jay's radio with a baseball bat, tore apart the cookbook, and burned his clothes with giddy zeal. She recounted one enactment of this ritual during which she set his work clothes ablaze: The sight of smoke and ash ascending into the sky far away from her home provided a visual representation of separation from Jay's malevolence. With his stinging voice more firmly ensconced in the past, a faint whisper of what once rung so loud, Priscilla was better able to enjoy warmhearted relationships with her children, her partner, her friends, and herself.

Priscilla's case exemplifies how the destruction of certain objects tied to an unhealthy relationship can establish symbolic distance from noxious remnants of the past. But an entirely different type of ritual can turn to concrete markers of actual distance to confirm separation from what came before and move forward less encumbered by ghosts. The physical setting of these personal grief rituals, the *where* of its design, often proves to be its most important element. Meaningful locations tied to past torments provide the most apt metaphor by which the bereaved can reaffirm a sense of measurable space apart from what must be left behind once and for all. One may visit a grave site to soothe themselves with a reminder that the deceased has been rendered harmless deep beneath the ground. Or the bereaved could say goodbye to a childhood home that need not be revisited ever again.

Kori long suspected that he never mourned his mother's death in full. An otherwise-happy and well-adjusted man in his early sixties who loved his job, his community, and his partner, he was saddled with the vague inkling that something remained unaddressed. We pondered over this peculiar impression that weighed on his mind twenty years after his mother died. Were there any feelings of grief left neglected? No. Kori openly expressed a full range of affect about the loss of his mother. Had his mother's lifelong disapproval of his vocation demoralized him, leading him to stymie his career? Not at all. He had sustained a successful career as an artist despite discouragements from his blue-collar siblings and parents. Perhaps he was replicating unhealthy relational dynamics between him and his mother in his fifteen-year marriage to his husband. Here, too, there were no clear signs of relational dysfunction.

I eventually shared my observation that Kori always raised concerns about unresolved mourning while talking about a recent visit to see one of his many doctors. Kori suffered numerous physical ailments as a child and continued to see a team of specialists throughout adulthood to manage chronic pain and the jumbled amalgam of symptoms that beleaguered his health. In his earliest years, being the sick child in the family invited his mother's scorn. She cast Kori as the object of her scorn, going so far as to ridicule him in front of his siblings. His brothers would sometimes take the reins, teasing Kori if ever he should complain about an upsurge of pain or opt to rest inside instead of playing outdoors with friends. He escaped his mother's wrath whenever he could by hiding beneath a thicket of cedar trees in the backyard, just far enough away from the house to monitor his mother's whereabouts safely from afar.

Now living in a world his mother no longer inhabited, she nonetheless managed to go on lambasting Kori. He harangued himself with charges of being "too sensitive." He brooded over the ways in which he should push himself to "get over" the pain and just "deal with it." When symptoms inevitably flared up, Kori belittled himself for being a "crybaby." This torrent of self-reproaches emerged with pronounced intensity each time he was en route to the psychiatrist, or the surgeon who operated on his wrist, or the chiropractor. In the shadow of otherwise-benevolent physicians, his mother loomed in expectations of belittling remarks.

This was the culprit that caused Kori to feel as if he were dwelling in a protracted state of mourning: He tiptoed through each day in anticipation of his mother and her cruelty lurking around every corner. Though he wrestled with guilt for wanting to be unburdened from her – "I feel like I should still *want* her to be here" – Kori was finally able to articulate his earnest wish to liberate himself from his mother, to move forward with a more secure sense of distance from his childhood. And from her. We began designing a personal grief ritual that guided him back to his hometown, halfway across the country, where he could destroy connections to the original source of his shame.

Kori decided that he would initiate his homecoming by revisiting the row of cedar trees that lined the far end of his childhood backyard. He used this as an opportunity to remind himself that his mother was no longer a threat and that he no longer needed to hide from his mother's cruel tauntings. Kori planned to then make his way to the nearby graveyard, where his mother was buried. He brought along a piece of paper and a pencil to create a stone *rubbing* – a basic printmaking technique that artists use to reproduce the texture of a surface – of her headstone. I asked Kori to describe the meaning behind this ritual, which I soon learned was twofold. First, incorporating artwork into its performance would be a confident gesture of defiance against his mother having discouraged him from pursuing the vocation he always desired. Second, Kori wanted to exert an ounce of aggression, too long directed towards himself, by tearing up a symbolic representation of her on his way out of town. Upon returning to Chicago, he shared how freeing it felt to toss shreds of his visit to her headstone into the wind. The tattered bits of paper whipped past his car as he drove out of town and into a future far away from his mother.

When the ritual must end

Grief rituals, like the very lives they aim to let go of, are destined to suffer a fate of growth and subsequent decay. Meaningful acts of mourning reach peak expression – a swell of woeful shouts and wailing, a resounding and passionate narrative recounting the deceased's life, or the red-hot crackling of a funeral pyre – then ebb in intensity until their performance is quiet and complete. As the ritual draws to a close, each participant is to fall silent in their grief and cease making purposeful noise. The traditional New Orleans jazz funeral begins with a second-line brass band playing soft and somber tones, then blasts forth in a jubilant fanfare of upbeat music to urge mourners into a raucous celebration of life; but in due time, a hush descends upon the parade as the musicians put down their instruments and the bereaved return home. The *after-tears* parties in modern-day South Africa pump out booming sounds of dance music until the inevitable moment when the last song has been played and the clinking of glasses decrescendos, signaling that it is time for tired partygoers to leave and seek rest. The fiery embers of the ritual ultimately cool into a heap of cold, gray cinders.

Grief itself may very well rise from the ashes and cry out once more for meaningful expression, but a time comes in which the formality of ritual is no longer needed to unearth feelings and thoughts about a loss. The journey through acute mourning arrives at a definitive end. The Malagasy of Madagascar, the Choctaw Native Americans of Oklahoma, and the Ifugao people of the Philippines all seem to understand that even the most prolonged liminal rituals are to be renounced in due time. Their use of double burials embodies patience alongside the eventual goal of no longer exhuming the dead. As the body is interred underground for the final time, forever out of sight and beyond reach, so too are scripted and structured acts of mourning buried for good.

From a clinical perspective, the formality of personal grief rituals should be abandoned when grief can be managed more spontaneously. The ritual is no longer needed when the bereaved individual has progressed through the ambiguities of liminality, separating themselves from the past and reincorporating themselves back into life after a death. Prescribed plans to mourn the dead become redundant when an array of affects can unfurl naturally, free from inhibition or emotional flooding. And the achievement of *absence-and-presence* allows one to, without targeted interventions, simultaneously let go of their previous bond while holding on to a symbolic and meaningful tie to the deceased if desired. Even those who struggle with an insecure attachment style, who err too strongly towards deactivation or hyperactivation of attachment behaviors in mourning, will have hopefully used personal grief rituals to usher in a more balanced expression of mourning and adaptation.

Ritual grows problematic when it becomes yet another compulsive routine devoid of the very thoughts and feelings it was originally intended to inspire. Reoccurring visits to the grave site find the bereaved staring blankly at their surrounds and whittling away time simply because they do not know what else to do with their day. An old photo album with pictures of the deceased is leafed through purely out of habit. Such stale ceremonialism is forever tempting the bereaved to step away from the difficult but rewarding work of being creative amid a new day and being attuned to one's present-day psychological needs. Acts of mourning that were once vibrant and full of meaning can degenerate into a half-hearted modus operandi, a familiar and comfortable pain that burrows deep into the psyche and requires excision. It is for this reason that cultural grief rituals crafted to meet its peoples' needs and systems of meaning at a specific moment eventually erode under the pressures of time and change, forcing humanity to abandon their tired and out-of-touch customs.

Psychotherapy itself can have this wearying nature over time. The bereaved client often shows up to their first few appointments and reports that the sheer act of being in the therapist's office gives pause to think and feel differently than they would have otherwise. But treatment can devolve into a dull drone, an unimaginative and repetitive procedure that no longer evokes new thoughts, affects, memories, or modes of relatedness. The same therapist who originally helped right the ship with a corrective personal grief ritual may need to call out to the bereaved, who now sails aimlessly about, and implore them to return to the shore.

Let us return once more to Matthew, who was discussed in previous chapters. He coped with the first anniversary of his sister's death by designing a personal grief ritual that helped him express emotions in a private and meaningful setting. He acknowledged the date for what it was, spent time with his wife and their two young children, and shared memories of the aunt they never got to meet. He would, over time, devise a separate ritual that helped him combat painful feelings of separation from his sister by planting sunflower seeds as she had always done.

The second anniversary of her death was fast approaching, and Matthew felt decidedly different about how he hoped to spend that day. His family was pushing through each holiday during the second year of his sister's absence in the same manner as the first year, with grave expressions on their faces and conversations that harped on past memories. Mourning, it seemed, had turned stagnant. Matthew grew tired of assuming a melancholic tone during every significant date on the calendar.

He and his wife continued to attend therapy together. During a session that was only a month away from the second anniversary, they hesitantly broached the topic of wanting to be excited about the future. They looked at me with timid expressions, like they were asking for me to approve of some mischievous plot. To their surprise, I enthusiastically invited them to consider how they might want to use the upcoming anniversary as a meaningful marker in time, as an opportunity to intentionally give greater focus towards what lay ahead, and to let themselves feel, as Matthew said, "anything at all that is positive or hopeful." Their shoulders lifted as they spoke with pride about their resiliency over the last two years. They had mourned with great sorrow and reverence, but the time had come to give greater energy towards new life. Their voices brimmed with lightness and relief as they made plans to take off work on the day of the second anniversary to spend the afternoon with their two children. They looked forward to enjoying a picnic and playing at their favorite nearby park in the city. Lastly, Matthew and his wife decided to share the exciting news with their children that they would soon have another little brother.

When cultural rituals fail to provide a meaningful avenue through mourning, each individual carries the potential to carve his or her own path by designing a personal grief ritual that guides the way towards a more authentic expression and experience of their loss. Nonetheless, the bereaved may find that their self-guided journey, once true in its course, has begun to lead them astray. The object of one's invention, the *personal sacred*, loses its luster. The ritual's effervescence fades away. Scheduling time to hold illusory conversations with the dead comes to lack its initial spark and vivacity. Revisiting a location tied to the lost relationship suddenly feels like an empty, affectless gesture.

While some make a point of backing away from the personal grief rituals they crafted, others find that their creations naturally fade out of mind over time. Grief and mourning emerge spontaneously and no longer require a cue. An unprompted cry of sorrow bellows forth when appropriate. The instinct to seek out continuing bonds becomes second nature. The bereaved forge new relationships, take part in novel activities, and open space within their home simply because they feel an intrinsic push to pursue a more robust life. Kendrick continued to listen to Jimi Hendrix, Cream, and Grateful Dead as a part of his daily life, though still with an occasional nod to his friend when a favorite song of theirs came on. Lucy attended baseball games across the country without feeling as if it were compulsory for her to draw out emotions about her father's absence during the seventh-inning stretch. And Kiara remained bound to her brother's symbolic presence, but without any conscious intention, like a healthy habit she no longer needed to will herself to do.

Those who stole away in quiet solitude to mourn the dead will do well to step back into the world of the living, a lively landscape replete with communal gatherings, social customs, and shared adventures to be had. A deep sense of belonging hopefully awaits on the other side of bereavement. Still, the individual will likely find that their passage through mourning has left an undying impression, an inextinguishable hunger for personal meaning and authentic emotional expression. Like the warm embrace of a mother or father eager to welcome us back home, one can always return to the secure base of a personal grief ritual to vent private feelings of joy and suffering, to walk and talk with the dead, or to say goodbye as many times as needed before once again venturing ahead into a future filled with more relationships whose absence will one day be mourned and whose presence may very well persist in spite of death.

References

Bowlby, J. (1963). Pathological mourning and childhood mourning. *Journal of the American Psychoanalytic Association, 11*, 500–541.

Conklin, B. A. (2007). Cannibalism and the work of culture in bereavement: Commentary on Gottlieb. *Journal of the American Psychoanalytic Association, 55*(4), 1253–1264.

Crowder, L. S. (2003). The Taoist (Chinese) way of death. In C. D. Bryant (Ed.), *Handbook of death & dying* (Vol. 2, pp. 673–686). Sage.

Cush, D., Robinson, C., & York, M. (2008). *Encyclopedia of Hinduism*. Routledge.

Goody, J. (1962). *Death, property, and the ancestors: A study of the mortuary customs of the LoDagaa of West Africa*. Tavistock Publications.

Herman, J. L. (1997). *Trauma and recovery*. Basic Books.

Holloway, A. (2014, February 15). Turning of the bones and the Madagascar dance with the dead. *Ancient Origins*. www.ancient-origins.net/ancient-places-africa/turning-bones-and-madagascar-dance-dead-001346

Hori, I. (1994). *Folk religion in Japan: Continuity and change*. Chicago University Press.

Isidro, M. C. (1978). Death in Baras. *Philippine Studies, 26*(4), 363–390.

Kidwell, C. S. (2007). *The Choctaws in Oklahoma: From tribe to nation, 1855–1970*. University of Oklahoma Press.

Kiong, T. C. (1990). Death rituals and ideas of pollution among the Chinese in Singapore. *Contributions to Southeast Asian Ethnography, 9*, 91–111.

Klein, M. (1940). Mourning and its relation to manic-depressive states. *The International Journal of Psychoanalysis, 21*, 125–153.

Kotze, E., Els, L., & Rajuili-Masilo, N. (2012). "Women . . . mourn and men carry on": African women storying mourning practices: A South African example. *Death Studies, 36*, 742–766.

Levine, E. (1997). Jewish views and customs on death. In P. Laungani & W. Young (Eds.), *Death and bereavement across cultures* (pp. 98–130). Routledge.

Mahler, M. S. (1972). On the first three subphases of the separation-individuation process. *The International Journal of Psychoanalysis, 53*(3), 333–338.

McGrath, P., & Phillips, E. (2008). Insights on end-of-life ceremonial practices of Australian Aboriginal peoples. *Collegian, 15*(4), 125–133.

Pliny the Younger. (1963). *The letters of the Younger Pliny* (B. Radice, Trans.). Penguin Books.
Prigerson, H. O., & Jacobs, S. C. (2001). Traumatic grief as a distinct disorder: A rationale, consensus criteria, and a preliminary empirical test. In M. S. Stroebe, R. O. Hansson, W. Stroebe, & H. Schut (Eds.), *Handbook of bereavement research: Consequences, coping, and care* (pp. 613–645). American Psychological Association.
Rank, O. (1945). *Will therapy and truth and reality*. Knopf.
Reeves, N. C. (2011). Death acceptance through ritual. *Death Studies, 35*(5), 408–419.
Santiago, L. P. R. (1993). The language of mourning and depression in Filipino and its Indonesian and Malayan cognates: Transcultural, sociological, historical, artistic, and therapeutic significance. *Philippine Quarterly of Culture and Society, 21*(3), 269–311.
Stroebe, M., Stroebe, W., van de Schoot, R., Schut, H., Abakoumkin, G., & Li, J. (2014). Guilt in bereavement: The role of self-blame and regret in coping with loss. *PLoS ONE, 9*(5), Article e96606. https://doi.org/10.1371/journal.pone.0096606
Van der Hart, O., & Ebbers, J. (1981). Rites of separation in strategic psychotherapy. *Psychotherapy: Theory, Research & Practice, 18*(2), 188–194.
Walker-Gillet, S. (2011). Death: Indigenous and western views. *Undergraduate Journal of Native Studies: Dbaajmowin, 1*, 83–102.
Watson, J. L. (1988). The structure of Chinese funerary rites: Elementary forms, ritual sequence, and the primacy of performance. In J. L. Watson & E. S. Rawski (Eds.), *Death ritual in late imperial and modern China* (pp. 3–19). University of California Press.
Weiss, J. (1993). *How psychotherapy works*. Guilford Press.
Worden, J. W. (2008). *Grief counseling and grief therapy: A handbook for the mental health practitioner* (4th ed.). Springer Publishing Company.
Yasien-Esmael, H., & Rubin, S. S. (2005). The meaning structures of Muslim bereavements in Israel: Religious traditions, mourning practices, and human experience. *Death Studies, 29*(6), 495–518.

Index

For Product Safety Concerns and Information please contact our EU representative GPSR@taylorandfrancis.com
Taylor & Francis Verlag GmbH, Kaufingerstraße 24, 80331 München, Germany

www.ingramcontent.com/pod-product-compliance
Ingram Content Group UK Ltd.
Pitfield, Milton Keynes, MK11 3LW, UK
UKHW020141200926
475702UK00005B/855
9780815384113